the **qigong** year

contents

introduction

Qigong is a self-healing art that originated in ancient China. It combines movement, meditation, and visualizations to maintain health; prevent and treat illness; reduce stress; and bring harmony to the mind, body, and spirit. The word qi (or ch'i) may be translated as "vital energy," and gong (or kung) means "skill," or to "exercise," "practice," or "refine." So qigong (ch'i kung) can be translated as "the skill, exercise, or cultivation of vital energy." The numerous systems of qigong, two of which are covered in depth in this book, share certain common elements: movement or posture; visualization; manipulation of the breath in prescribed ways, as well as the maintenance of natural breathing; and meditation following periods of exercise.

Practicing qigong regularly can improve your general well-being and balance your physical and mental health. It energizes the blood and internal organs, which leaves you feeling refreshed and invigorated. The more you practice qigong, the more qi you will have within your system and the more energetic you will feel. The exercises help make your body stronger and more supple, improve your posture, align your spine, and relax your shoulder and neck muscles. The psychological benefits are far-reaching—qigong can help stabilize your moods so that you are better able to deal with life's challenges.

This book is designed for you to work through on a month-by-month basis. You may read through the entire book before starting, but it's not necessary.

Set aside between 10 and 30 minutes for each exercise session. Read all of the exercises and theory for each month before you start your practice. Follow the instructions very carefully and perfect the exercise over several days. Only once you feel completely comfortable with a qigong exercise should you proceed to the next one. It is much better for you to learn a few exercises at a deep level than to learn all the exercises at a lower level. After the physical exercise, spend time on a meditation that appeals to you and suits your needs; again, anywhere from 10 to 30 minutes is appropriate.

before you start

- Wear loose clothing so that you can stretch and move freely.
- Choose a suitable place, either indoors or outdoors. Ideally, it should be quiet, with a good flow of fresh air but sheltered from the wind. If you are indoors, open a window to allow the elements in (unless there is a storm outside). Practice away from pollution (such as traffic fumes or radiation from electrical equipment).
- Keep your mind calm before and during the exercises. Do not practice if you are highly stressed, grieving, or very emotional.
- Be mindful of your entire body. Try to be aware of the position of your limbs, hands and feet, back, torso, and all your joints.
- Try to do the exercises in a relaxed manner without any force (unless specified) or stiffness. Aim to make your movements smooth, gentle, and deliberate. Smooth, coordinated movements enable qi to circulate freely throughout your body.
- Do not practice after drinking alcohol or smoking, or within a half-hour of a meal.
- If you are taking medication, seek your doctor's advice before starting a qigong practice.
- If you find yourself upset or distracted during practice, it's often better to stop the exercise, rub your body down (see the meditation sections), and find another time or place to continue.

general caution

There are no particular health restrictions for practicing qigong, but if you suffer from a medical condition, seek your doctor's advice before you begin. Once you do start, proceed slowly.

Perform the qigong exercises and meditations in a relaxed, natural way, listening to your body and not extending beyond your limits. Don't force yourself to continue with an exercise if you begin to feel strained or uncomfortable.

Women can continue their practice during menstruation. In fact, since qigong aids circulation, moodiness, cramps, and headaches, menstruating women will benefit from its practice. Women who have heavy periods should not bring their energies to the lower Dan Tian, which is just below the navel, but should instead concentrate on the solar plexus.

Qigong exercises can also be practiced during pregnancy. However, pregnant women should be sensible and not overdo the very active movements. The meditations provide a good flow of qi, which is essential for growth and can help strengthen the bond between mother and baby.

introducing ba duan jin

For the first eight months you will be learning Ba Duan Jin (Eight Pieces of Brocade), a basic form of qigong related to a style taught by the Bodhidharma (the originator of Zen Buddhism) to Shaolin monks in the 6th century CE. The individual exercises that make up this form are inscribed on the walls of the Shaolin monastery. The monks there continue to practice it on a daily basis to maintain their health and strengthen their vital energy.

The dynamic exercises that make up the Ba Duan Jin form are very popular and, being simple, ideal for beginners. They are more than merely physical exercises—like all forms of qigong, the techniques are designed to improve the amount or flow of qi (vital energy) in your body. Only by involving your mind in your qigong practice will you gain the full benefit of the exercises. But, even as simple physical exercises, the Ba Duan Jin routines will loosen muscles, improve posture, enhance blood circulation, and promote relaxation.

spring

beginnings

Spring is the time of new beginnings, when animals emerge from their hibernation burrows and winter hideouts with renewed energy and vitality, eager for what lies ahead of them. The start of a new year is also a good time to realize the latent potential of our bodies and minds. This is a great time to give your body a thorough "spring cleaning" and start to awaken the flow of qi within your being, filling your lungs and every cell in your body with fresh vitality. A firm resolution to commit yourself to qigong will bring your mind, body, and spirit back in harmony with nature, making you more healthy, happy, and peaceful.

month 1
month 2
month 3

month 1

What is in the end to be shrunken, begins
   by first being stretched out.
What is in the end to be weakened, begins by
   first being made strong.
What is in the end to be thrown down, begins
   by first being set high.
What is in the end to be despoiled, begins by
   first being richly endowed.
Herein is the subtle wisdom of life. The soft
   and weak overcome the hard and strong.
Just as the fish must not leave the deeps, so
   the ruler must not display his weapons.

from the *Tao Te Ching*

contents:

Stretching helps energy begin flowing around your body.

The first month of spring is a time of new beginnings. To make a good start to your spring, you need to shake off winter's apathy and stretch your body, awakening the flow of qi so that you can become truly revitalized, relaxed and ready for what lies ahead.

This month, you will learn the first of eight exercises from the Ba Duan Jin (Eight Pieces of Brocade or Eight Fine Exercises) form of qigong. This exercise, called Holding the Heavens, stretches and reinvigorates the body. The exercise brings to the mind an image of a cat stretching. If you watch a cat that has just woken up, you'll notice that it never gets up and starts walking immediately. First, it stretches and preens itself. This may well have been the inspiration that led the ancient Chinese to develop this exercise—it is the perfect way to help yourself feel awake and revitalized in the morning.

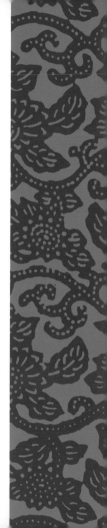

❹ Exhale, bringing your arms down in a circular motion and lowering your heels. Coordinate your breathing so that you complete your exhalation as your arms return to their starting position by your sides. Repeat up to 9 times.

Keep your fingers interlaced and keep your arms fully extended as you push up to the heavens.

Your heels should lift from the ground at the same time as your arms reach their fullest stretch.

holding the heavens

Once you have mastered the basic exercise, you may proceed to the advanced form.

❶ Stand with your back straight, your legs together, and your arms at your sides with your palms facing inward and lightly touching your sides. Look straight ahead.

❷ Take a step to the left. Your feet should now be shoulder-width apart. Bend your knees while maintaining a straight back so that your torso moves downward, as though you were riding a horse. This position is called the Horse Riding Stance. Be gentle on yourself, and don't bend your knees at an angle greater than 45 degrees. As you become more proficient with this posture, you'll find that your knees will naturally bend more.

❸ Giving it your full attention, lift your hands to the sides of your head and bring them to eye level, with your fingertips touching your temples slightly above and in front of your ears. Keep your fingers extended with your palms facing the ground.

❹ Lower your hands to chest level. Turn your palms so that they face each other with 4 inches (10 cm) between them.

❺ Rotate your hands so that your palms face upward. Your fingers should still be extended, but bring your fingertips together until they touch.

❻ Bend forward from the waist, place the backs of your hands flat on the ground, and push downward. If you cannot comfortably reach this far, let your hands hover (see illustration).

The backs of your hands should be parallel to the ground as you push downward. Listen to your body and go as far down as is comfortable.

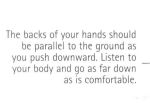

❼ Now lift your hands a little and rotate your arms, turning your elbows outward so that your palms face forward.

❽ Clench your fists. Keeping your back straight, begin to raise your torso back to a vertical position, lifting from the waist. As your body straightens, extend your elbows and straighten your arms (see illustration on page 21).

❾ Your torso should now be vertical. Bend your elbows and raise your arms and fists to chest height. Your elbows should be pointing out to your sides, with your fists facing each other and separated by 4 to 5 inches (10 to 12 cm).

❿ Open your fists so that your palms face downward.

⓫ Rotate your hands so that your palms face upward and push them above your head with force. Your elbows should remain slightly bent so that your arms form a circle around your head. While carrying out this movement, keep your eyes on your fingertips.

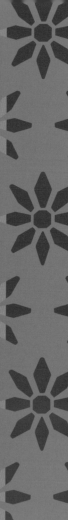

⑫ Lower your arms so that they hang by your sides, with your palms facing inward. Your hands may lightly touch your sides.

⑬ Remain in the Horse Riding Stance for a few seconds. Repeat the exercise up to 9 times. When you have finished the repetitions, straighten your body and return to the starting position. If you find doing many repetitions uncomfortable, build up slowly from fewer repetitions.

With your fists still clenched, pull your upper body up slowly and deliberately, taking care to keep your back straight.

holding the heavens

As with the other Ba Duan Jin routines, this exercise has a seated version. The seated version is particularly suitable for the elderly and for those who need to progress more gently.

❶ Sit comfortably on the ground or on a chair. Keep your back straight.

❷ Raise your arms above your head so that they are vertical, with your palms facing downward.

❸ Interlace your fingers and rotate your palms to face upward.

❹ While inhaling, push upward with your palms, keeping your fingers interlaced. Straighten your elbows and fully extend your arms (see illustration).

❺ Without lifting your body from the ground, try to stretch your torso and pull in your stomach.

❻ Exhale and relax, lowering your hands to just above your head, with your palms facing down. Repeat up to 9 times.

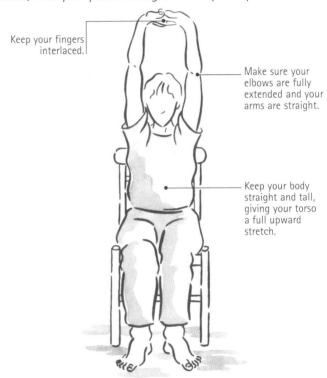

Keep your fingers interlaced.

Make sure your elbows are fully extended and your arms are straight.

Keep your body straight and tall, giving your torso a full upward stretch.

mastering the life force

According to ancient Chinese beliefs, air is vital energy in and of itself. To breathe is to inhale the life force, so it is essential that you know how to breathe properly. This may sound strange—breathing is, after all, a natural, automatic process. But very few of us truly breathe properly. When you inhale shallowly, an insufficient amount of oxygen reaches your body. When you do not fully exhale, you do not completely excrete the waste products of respiration (carbon dioxide). Babies naturally breathe from the bottom of their lungs, using their diaphragms to fully inhale and exhale. But as we become older, we tend to breathe from higher up in our lungs or even from our throats.

So what is correct breathing? Each form of exercise or spiritual practice has its own methods; the type that you will learn as part of your qigong practice is called abdominal breathing. As its name implies, this means breathing from your abdomen. Although it is the lungs that fill with air, the mechanism of breathing involves the entire chest and abdomen—in particular, the diaphragm. According to Chinese theory, the energy associated with breathing should circulate back and forth between the abdomen and the nose.

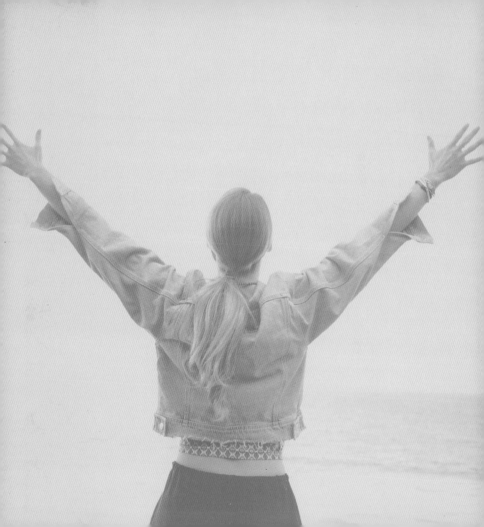

abdominal breathing: lying down

Here is one simple method of abdominal breathing:

❶ Lie on your back on the floor with your hands by your sides. You may place a pillow under your head, if you wish.

❷ Bring your attention to your abdomen. You will quickly become aware of its natural rise and fall.

❸ You should enter a state of deep relaxation. You may even fall asleep, but as your power of concentration increases, you will be able to remain awake throughout.

❹ Place your left hand on your stomach and your right palm on top of it. Remain like this for a few minutes, letting your body's natural rhythms guide your breathing.

❺ When you feel that you have relaxed and recharged yourself with vital energy, slowly get up. Stay quiet for a minute or two—this gives you time to adjust.

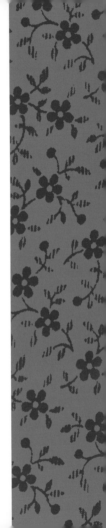

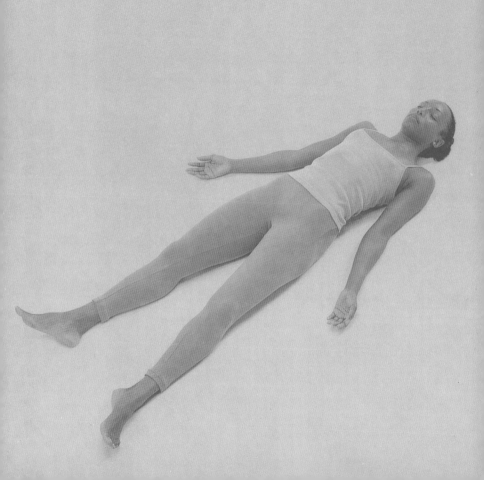

month2

The Tao is like an empty bowl, which in being
  used can never fill up.
Fathomless, it seems to be the origin of all
  things.
It blunts all sharp edges; it unties all tangles;
It harmonizes all lights; it unites the world into
  one whole.
Hidden in the deeps
Yet it seems to exist forever. I do not know
  whose child it is.
It seems to be the common ancestor of all, the
  father of things.

from the *Tao Te Ching*

contents:

Increasing your body's ability to take in qi is vital for health and spiritual growth.

In the first month, you learned how to stretch your body and fill it with vital energy. During the second month, you will build on what you've learned so far and increase your body's ability to take in qi by exercising your lungs.

The second Ba Duan Jin exercise, Drawing the Bow, increases your ability to absorb qi and helps move it around your body, making your entire body, and particularly your chest, healthier. It opens up your chest and increases the vital capacity of your lungs. In addition to physically strengthening the lungs, the deep breathing associated with the exercise also promotes efficient gaseous exchange within the lungs. Drawing the Bow is particularly helpful for ailments associated with the chest. If you have asthma or other breathing difficulties, practicing the exercise regularly can bring you relief. Drawing the Bow also strengthens the muscles of your chest, back, and arms. If you do the exercise in the Horse Riding Stance, you will find that your legs and buttocks are also strengthened.

In this chapter you will also learn about the three Dan Tians, the main concentration points in the body for qi, and the Microcosmic Circle, which is a way for qi to flow around the body. There is also a further abdominal breathing exercise, this time performed in a seated position, which enables you to fill your abdomen with qi.

This month also contains the first meditation of the book, a simple counting meditation that helps you clear your mind and cultivate qi. This helps to highlight the difference between the two main ways of practicing qigong; active qigong takes place during the physical qigong exercises, while passive qigong manifests itself during any type of meditation.

Qigong has much to offer, but these gifts come only with regular practice. Try to incorporate qigong into your daily life and you will reap the benefits.

drawing the bow

The aim of this exercise is to move vital energy around your body. While performing the exercise, you'll find it is helpful to imagine that you are actually drawing a bow to shoot an arrow. Visualizing a circular target for the arrow will improve your concentration.

❶ Stand with your feet shoulder-width apart and bend your knees. Lower your torso into the Horse Riding Stance.

❷ Cross your arms in front of your chest with the left arm tucked under the right and your open palms facing your chest. Point the index finger of your right hand and bend the other fingers into the palm. Make your left hand into a loose fist, with your thumb touching the tip of your index finger (see illustration).

❸ Extend your right arm, pointing to the right with your index finger. Follow your right hand with your eyes.

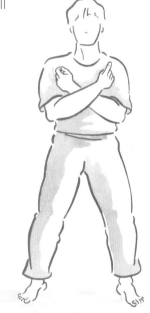

❹ At the same time, draw your left arm back with your elbow bent at shoulder height, as if you were pulling back the string of the bow. Your left elbow should point in the opposite direction of your right hand (see illustration).

❺ Breathe in deeply as you pull back on the bowstring. As you exhale, mentally release the arrow and relax your arms out of the stretch.

❻ After releasing the arrow, come up from the Horse Riding Stance and rise to a full standing position. Then repeat, this time shooting to your left side. Repeat the exercise up to 9 times on each side.

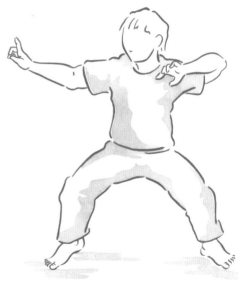

drawing the bow

Once you have mastered the initial technique, you can take the exercise of Drawing the Bow a step further.

❶ Stand with your back straight, your legs together, and your arms at your sides with your palms inward and lightly touching your sides. Look straight ahead.

❷ Take a step to the left. Your feet should be shoulder-width apart. Lower yourself into the Horse Riding Stance.

❸ Clench both fists. Hold your right fist about 1 foot (30 cm) in front of your eyes and your left fist by your right shoulder, as if you were boxing against a tall opponent. Keep your eyes on your right fist.

❹ Fully extend your right arm out to your right side and point your left elbow out to your left, again as if you were drawing a bow (see illustration). Both fists should be at shoulder level. You should be aiming for a wider stretch than in the basic technique, with your chest fully open.

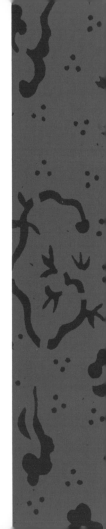

❺ Slowly turn your head to look first to the right and then to the left.

❻ Reverse the position of your fists—hold your left fist about 1 foot (30 cm) in front of your eyes and your right fist by your left shoulder. Return to the Horse Riding Stance and repeat the exercise on the left side of your body.

❼ Return to the initial position and repeat the exercise a total of 9 times on each side. If you find doing so many repetitions uncomfortable, aim to build up slowly from fewer repetitions.

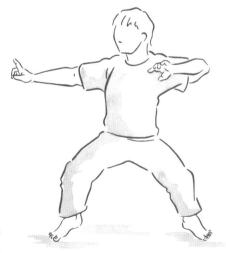

drawing the bow

This exercise can also be done while in a seated position. Ideally, it should be carried out in either a full lotus or a half lotus position. However, any position in which you are comfortable and your back is straight is fine.

❶ Sit comfortably with a straight back.

❷ Cross your arms in front of your chest, with your right arm under your left and your palms facing your chest.

❸ Imagine that you are drawing a bow to shoot an arrow to the left. Fully extend your left arm, pointing to your left with the first finger and bending the other fingers of your left hand into your palm. Follow the path of your left hand with your eyes.

❹ At the same time, draw your right arm back with your elbow bent at shoulder height, as if you were pulling back the string of the bow. Your right elbow should point in the opposite direction of your left hand (see illustration).

❺ Breathe in deeply as you pull back on the bowstring. As you exhale, mentally release the arrow and relax your arms out of the stretch.

❻ Repeat the exercise, this time shooting to your right side. Repeat the exercise a total of 9 times on each side.

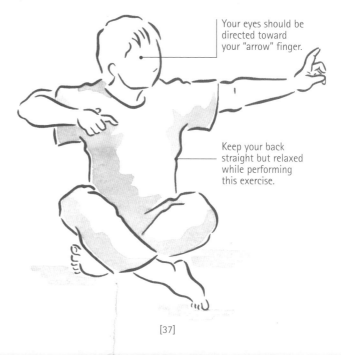

Your eyes should be directed toward your "arrow" finger.

Keep your back straight but relaxed while performing this exercise.

the three dan tians

There are three important points in the body that are particularly suited to meditation. They are known as the Dan Tians. Dan means "crystal" or the "essence of energy," while Tian means "field" or "area for the essence of energy."

The first point, called the upper Dan Tian, or the third eye, is between the eyebrows. The second point, the middle Dan Tian, is at the solar plexus. You can energize your entire body by bringing your attention to the middle Dan Tian. When you are stressed or feel under pressure, this is the area that may feel tight or knotted. The third point, or lower Dan Tian, is at a point 1½ inches (4 cm) below the navel.

The Dan Tians store qi. Initially, stored qi flows around your body like a gas, causing sensations such as warmth or tingling. As you continue to practice qigong, the nature and sensations of qi change to become liquid. As a result, you may feel warmth like that of blood or milk from a nursing mother. With continued practice, the energy transforms once again into crystal (Dan). When a Buddhist monk who has achieved a high level of enlightenment dies and is cremated, crystals, called Xie Li Zi, may be found in his ashes.

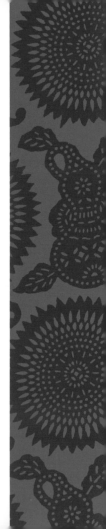

When you first practice qigong, you focus on bringing qi to the lower Dan Tian. You may feel tingling there. With continued practice, qi rises through the Ren Channel at the front of the body, passes through the solar plexus, the third eye, and over the crown, and then returns down the Du Channel at the back of the body. This circle is known as the Microcosmic Circle. The tip of your tongue must touch your upper palate behind your teeth in order for qi to flow around the Microcosmic Circle. Eventually, the Microcosmic Circle will become clear, making you strong and healthy.

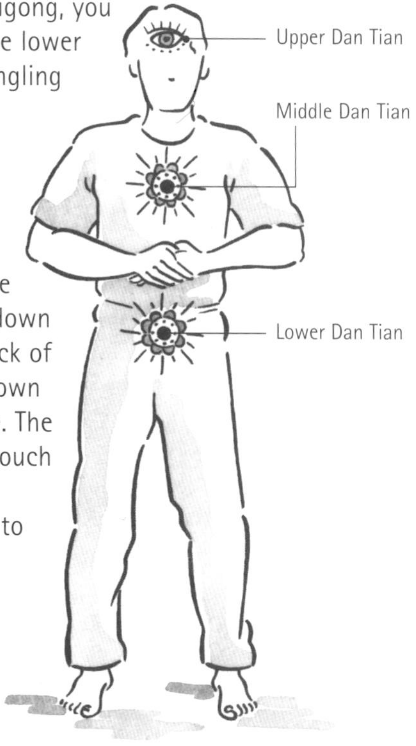

Upper Dan Tian

Middle Dan Tian

Lower Dan Tian

abdominal breathing: sitting

The next variation of abdominal breathing involves performing the exercise in a seated posture:

❶ Sit cross-legged on the floor with your back reasonably straight. If you find it difficult to sit on the floor, you may sit on a chair. If you do decide to use a chair, try to sit on the edge of the seat, because this position encourages you to keep your back straight.

❷ Place your left palm on your stomach and your right palm over your left hand. Become aware of your breathing. Follow your breath as it flows in and out of your nostrils without trying to alter its natural rhythm. As you become more relaxed, your breathing will become deeper.

❸ After about 5 minutes, start following the inhaled breath all the way to your abdomen; similarly, follow the exhaled

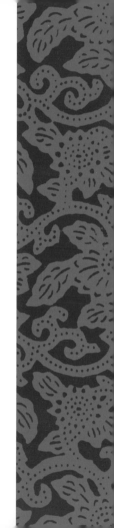

breath from your abdomen to your nostrils. Always remain aware of the rise and fall of your abdomen as you follow the breath. If you lose concentration or your thoughts begin to wander, gently steer your mind back to your breathing.

❹ As you progress, you may begin to detect an inner glow coming from your abdomen. At first, you may think that it's just your imagination, but the glow will develop until your whole abdomen becomes unmistakably warm. This is a sign of good progress in your practice. According to ancient theory, it signifies that the abdomen is filling with qi. Once you have developed this sensation, you can circulate the qi to your internal organs or limbs as a form of self-healing or to assist in physical activities.

You can also perform this breathing exercise while standing. This has the advantage of strengthening your kidneys and legs and developing your capacity to connect with the earth's energy. You will begin to feel distinctly rooted to the ground—a very pleasant experience.

counting meditation 1

Having mastered the abdominal breathing technique, you may now move on to the next level. This exercise is also practiced lying down, and it involves counting your inhalations and exhalations. One inhalation and one exhalation are counted as one whole breath. At first, start with 25 breaths, and then increase to 50, 75, and, ultimately, 100 breaths.

Initially, you may find that you become so relaxed that you lose count of the number of breaths, but eventually you will be able to count up to 100 breaths. When you reach that stage, your power of concentration will have improved greatly. But even if you do lose count and fall asleep during the exercise, you are still benefiting from the deep state of relaxation that you have achieved.

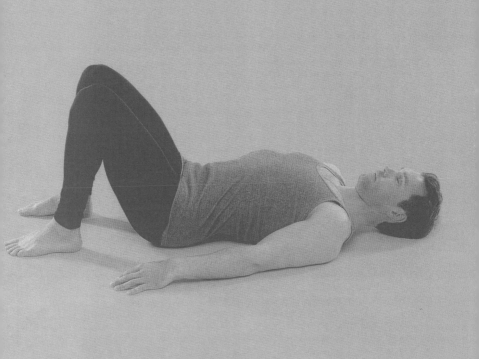

month3

Between Heaven and Earth, there seems to be a
    bellows:
It is empty, and yet it is inexhaustible;
The more it works, the more comes out of it.
No amount of words can fathom it:
Better look for it within you.

from the *Tao Te Ching*

contents:

Growth involves filling your body with different energies so that your own energy can expand and develop.

The third month, late spring, is a time of increased growth, a time for obtaining energy from the elements and transforming it into useful forms, readying yourself for the burst of summer growth.

This month, you will learn how to use different energies for your benefit, how to nurture those energies, and how to let them flow throughout your body to recharge it. In addition, you will learn about how two forms of qi, prenatal and postnatal, are obtained.

You will be introduced to the third Ba Duan Jin exercise, Separating Heaven and Earth, which harnesses the energies of heaven and earth to give your body a full lateral stretch,

energizing your entire torso and leaving it open and relaxed. This exercise helps you obtain energy more efficiently from your food and is particularly beneficial for digestive disorders. According to the ancient Chinese, it stimulates two key meridians—that of the stomach and that of the spleen. The stomach meridian is the energetic pathway that has the stomach as its root organ. If you suffer from indigestion, stomach ulcers, constipation, or diarrhea, this exercise will be helpful through its effect on the stomach meridian. In addition, many meridians run through the center of the body, so the exercise will also benefit a range of other conditions.

The sitting variation of Separating Heaven and Earth, in addition to the benefits described above, strengthens the neck muscles and aids blood circulation, especially in the neck and head areas.

Two new abdominal breathing exercises are introduced. Both exercises are helpful if you suffer from high blood pressure, and they also enable you to establish a more grounded relationship with the earth.

separating heaven and earth

In this exercise, one hand pushes up to the sky while the other pushes down to the ground, hence the name Separating Heaven and Earth. You will obtain the greatest benefit from this exercise if, while your arms are fully extended, you let yourself feel the energy of the heavens flowing into your body through your upstretched arm and the energy of the earth entering your body through your downstretched arm. This influx of energy will invigorate the middle of your body—your torso.

❶ Stand with your feet shoulder-width apart, with your feet facing forward and your arms hanging at your sides. Look straight ahead.

❷ Place your hands together in front of your abdomen with your palms horizontal and facing each other, left palm on top of the right, as though you were holding a ball. Inhale deeply, imagining that you are inhaling golden light or healing energy.

❸ Raise your left arm above your head so that it is fully extended. Drop your right arm down by your side. Imagine that your arms are the hands of a clock. If viewed from the front, your left arm would be at "one o'clock" and your right arm would be at "seven o'clock." Your left palm should face the heavens and your right palm should face the earth (see illustration). Exhale deeply.

❹ Fully extend your arms until you feel a nice stretch.

❺ Repeat the exercise a total of 9 times on each side of the body.

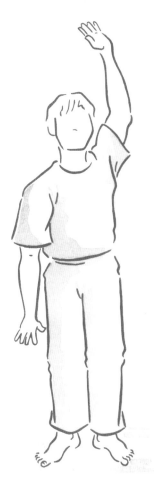

separating heaven and earth

Here is a more advanced form of the exercise:

❶ Stand with your legs together and your back straight. Let your arms hang down with your palms lightly touching your sides; look straight ahead.

❷ Take a step to the left. Lower yourself into the Horse Riding Stance, keeping your arms hanging by your sides so that your palms now gently touch your knees.

❸ From your waist, rotate your body to the left, straightening out your left leg in front of you as you turn. Your right leg should remain bent at the knee.

❹ Raise your left hand to face level, making a fist about 1 foot (30 cm) in front of your eyes, with your palm facing toward your face. Raise your right hand to waist level, keep your elbow bent at a 90-degree-angle, and make a fist with your palm facing upward. Keep your eyes on your left fist (see illustration).

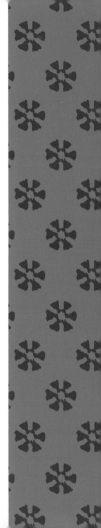

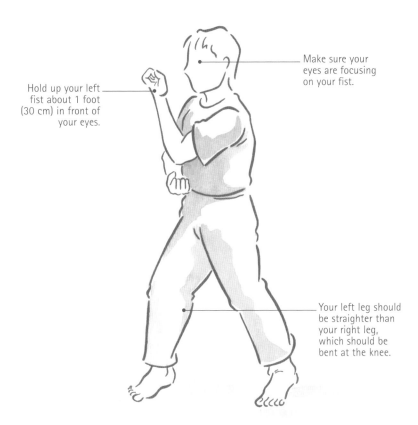

Hold up your left fist about 1 foot (30 cm) in front of your eyes.

Make sure your eyes are focusing on your fist.

Your left leg should be straighter than your right leg, which should be bent at the knee.

❺ Bend forward from your waist. Touch your left fist to your right foot, keeping your right fist at waist level. You should still be looking at your left hand (see illustration).

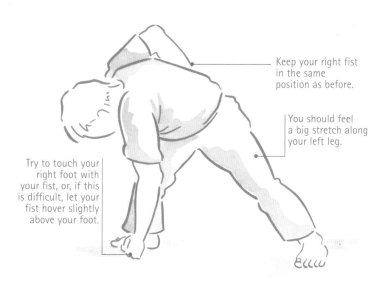

Keep your right fist in the same position as before.

You should feel a big stretch along your left leg.

Try to touch your right foot with your fist, or, if this is difficult, let your fist hover slightly above your foot.

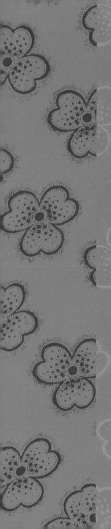

❻ Straightening from your waist, raise your torso and rotate to the left. Look to the left. As you move your upper body, straighten your right leg and let your left knee bend.

❼ Bring your left arm up with your elbow bent so that the fingers of your left hand point to your eyes and nose and your palm faces up. Your right hand should be at waist level, with your palm facing up.

❽ With your left palm still facing up, push your left hand up above your head as if shielding your eyes from the sun.

❾ Keeping your eyes on your left hand, press downward with your right hand. Stretch toward your right leg but don't touch it. This will give you a sideways stretch.

❿ Return to the Horse Riding Stance and repeat the exercise on the other side. You may repeat the entire routine up to 9 times on each side, but build up gradually if you feel tired or strained. At the end of the session, go back to the Horse Riding Stance, then stand up straight with your legs together and look straight ahead.

separating heaven and earth

You can also perform the routine sitting down. However, this version of the exercise is not recommended if you have high blood pressure.

❶ Sit comfortably with your back straight.

❷ Hold your hands with your fingers interlaced behind your head. Your palms should touch your head.

❸ Lean your head back. Breathe in and look up while pressing your hands forward. Breathe out and look down.

❹ Breathe in, turn your head and eyes to the right and press your hands to the left (see illustration). Repeat on the other side, breathing out as you smoothly turn your head to the left and press your hands to the right.

❺ Repeat the entire routine a total of 9 times on both sides of your body.

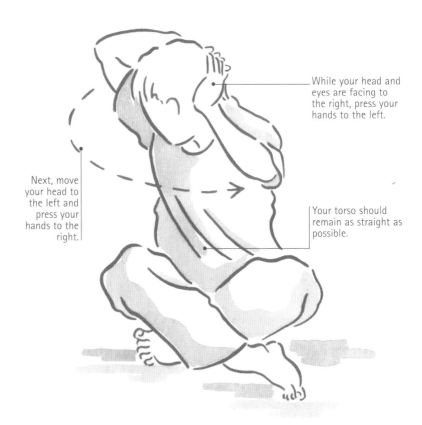

While your head and eyes are facing to the right, press your hands to the left.

Next, move your head to the left and press your hands to the right.

Your torso should remain as straight as possible.

abdominal breathing: standing

The standing version of abdominal breathing is a basic part of the practice known as rooting, in which advanced martial artists demonstrate their ability to remain standing while strong men attempt to push them to the floor.

❶ Stand with your feet parallel and shoulder-width apart. Make a concentrated effort to feel the ground beneath your feet. Lean forward slightly on the balls of your feet.

❷ Looking straight ahead, bend your knees slightly. To help keep your back straight, imagine a thread connecting the top of your head to the sky. Your head should be slightly lowered—this ensures that there is a straight line from the base of your spine to the top of your head (see illustration).

❸ Close your eyes. Let your arms hang loosely at your sides with your palms facing inward. Stand in this position for about 5 minutes. Periodically check to ensure that your body is not holding any tension. If you feel tension, tense and then relax that part of your body. By doing this, you should be able to get your entire body to relax.

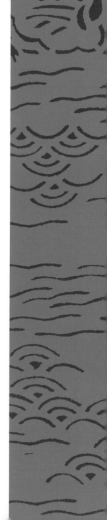

❹ To start abdominal breathing, bring your attention to your abdomen and concentrate on it for a few minutes.

❺ Become aware of the natural up and down motion of your abdomen as you breathe, but don't try to control or alter this motion—just breathe naturally.

❻ Enhance your concentration by adding a visualization exercise. As you breathe in, imagine golden light filling your abdomen. As you breathe out, imagine that you are exhaling black smoke; feel all tension being expelled from your body. Initially, do this exercise for 10 minutes, then build up to 20 minutes. As you stand rooted to the ground, exchanging bad energy for good, you resemble a tree drawing nourishment from the earth and the heavens.

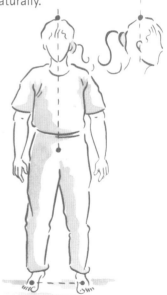

concentrating on the center

Close your abdominal breathing routine with this exercise:

❶ Place your hands on top of each other just below your navel (see illustration).

❷ Be aware of sensations, such warmth or tingling, in the area of your belly as it is nourished with qi. You may not feel anything, but if you do feel something, try to concentrate on it fully. Maintain this position for a few minutes.

❸ Now rub your hands together. Rub your face gently. You can also rub down the rest of your body.

As you practice standing abdominal breathing, you may have some interesting sensations. Make a note of your experiences in a diary. Having a record of your daily progress is very encouraging and it will help you stay motivated to practice.

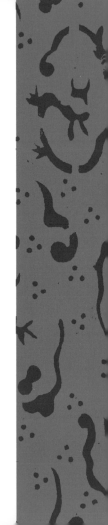

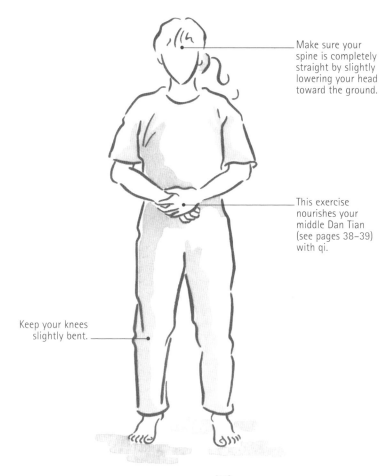

Make sure your spine is completely straight by slightly lowering your head toward the ground.

This exercise nourishes your middle Dan Tian (see pages 38–39) with qi.

Keep your knees slightly bent.

prenatal and postnatal qi

Qi, or vital energy, drives the entire universe, not just the human body. The Huangdi Neijing (The Yellow Emperor's Canon of Internal Medicine), a text written for the Yellow Emperor in the eighth century BCE, describes two basic types of qi within the body: prenatal qi and postnatal qi.

Prenatal, or original, qi is an inner driving energy that is given to you by your parents—yang energy comes from your father and yin energy comes from your mother. These two energies fuse to create prenatal qi. Prenatal energy is stored deep inside your body. Your physical structure and your basic physiology—whether you are strong and healthy or suffer from health problems—are all due to the type of prenatal energy inherited from your parents.

Postnatal qi is what you rely on to continue to stay alive after birth; it is derived from the food and water you eat and drink, the air you breathe, and the regeneration you gain during sleep. Postnatal qi is related to the 12 primary meridians in the body and their associated organs. Prenatal and postnatal qi act and rely upon each other; together they form the "true qi" of the body—the source of energy used in daily life.

Although food, water, air, and sleep are sources of postnatal qi, acquiring this qi also uses energy. For example, you need to expend

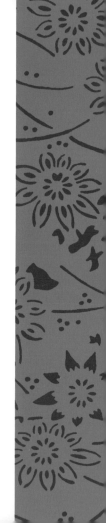

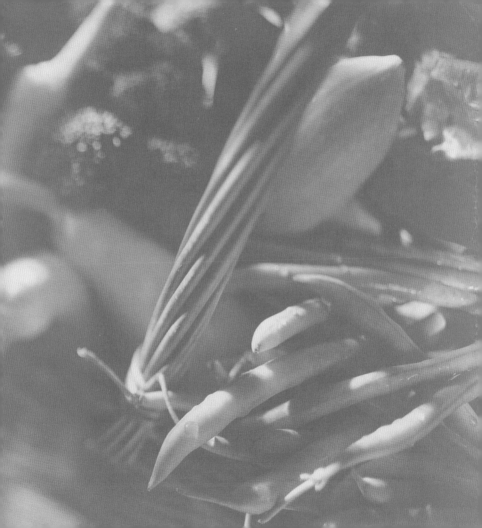

energy to digest food and eliminate wastes, which is why you often feel tired immediately after eating. While breathing, you expend energy separating pollutants from air to obtain clean oxygen. In a poorly ventilated room, you will soon start to yawn in an effort to obtain fresh air, and you may also feel sleepy or even faint.

Sleep also uses energy. Have you ever woken up in the morning and still felt tired? Just as with breathing, there are different ways of sleeping—some of which are regenerative and some of which are not so beneficial. Even though you are asleep, your brain may still be active, dreaming or dwelling on stressful thoughts, and thus using energy. If you sleep in an awkward position, qi will not flow easily around your body and you'll feel stiff in the morning.

Qigong was developed to specifically impact prenatal and postnatal qi, to balance and enhance true qi for health and longevity, and to direct energy to spiritual development. All of these energies direct our life activities and link us to the divine.

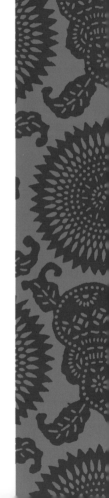

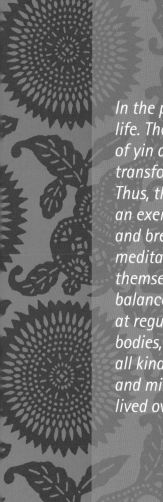

In the past, people practiced the Tao, the way of life. They understood the principle of balance, of yin and yang, as represented by the transformation of the energies of the universe. Thus, they formulated practices such as Tao-in, an exercise combining stretching, massaging, and breathing to promote energy flow, and meditation to help maintain and harmonize themselves with the universe. They ate a balanced diet at regular times, arose and retired at regular hours, avoided overstressing their bodies, and refrained from over-indulgence of all kinds. They maintained well-being of body and mind; thus, it is not surprising that they lived over one hundred years.

from the *Huangdi Neijing*

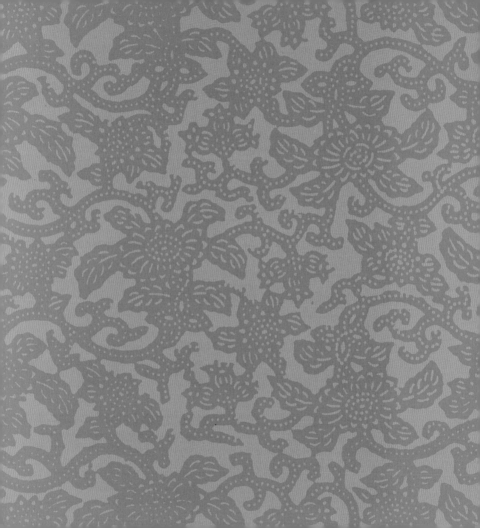

summer

growth

Summer is the time when seeds planted in the spring start to reveal some of their future potential, when flowers come out and show their true beauty. In your qigong practice, you too will have grown, in your own way and at your own rate. What is important is that a change is taking place, however slowly it is happening. In this season, you will learn how the five elements that make up nature and our very bodies can be used to bring us back into harmony in a pleasant and relaxing way.

month 4
month 5
month 6

month4

The Spirit of the Fountain dies not. It is called the
  Mysterious Feminine.
The doorway of the Mysterious Feminine is called
  the root of Heaven and Earth.
Lingering like gossamer, it has only a hint of
  existence;
And yet when you draw upon it, it is
  inexhaustible.

from the *Tao Te Ching*

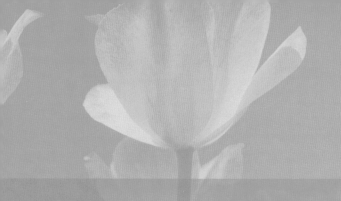

contents:

Using the energies of nature's Five Elements strengthens your mind and body.

The fourth month is the month when flowers come into bloom, when spring gradually gives way to summer. It is a time when increased light and warmth bring us fully into the outdoor world, allowing us to absorb the many energies the universe has to offer.

The Ba Duan Jin exercise of Looking Backward, in both the basic and advanced versions, is a boon for anyone who suffers from back problems. Regular practice increases the flexibility of the spine. According to ancient Chinese thought, a supple spine is indicative of life and youth, while a stiff spine is associated with death and old age. Moreover, the benefits to the spine in turn convey benefits to other parts of the body; the spinal column contains the spinal cord, and spinal nerves emerge along the length of the

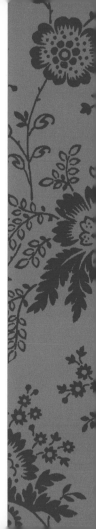

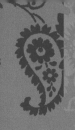

spinal cord, branching out to various organs. This exercise helps keep that part of the nervous system healthy. In addition, it nourishes the internal organs with vital energy and freshly oxygenated blood, increases circulation to the brain, and helps to relieve headaches.

The sitting variation of the exercise strengthens and increases the flexibility of your head, neck, and waist muscles. It also gently massages the internal organs and enhances blood circulation.

This month, you will be introduced to the Five Elements in nature, and how their energies affect your physical and emotional well-being. You will also see how meditating on the individual elements can bring relief to specific ailments and can also give a general sense of exhilaration and well-being. The first of the five Meditations on the Elements featured in this book is a Meditation on Water, which can be particularly helpful if you suffer from lower back problems, a lack of vitality, or fearfulness. In a sense, meditating on water can help to wash away your fears and difficulties, leaving you refreshed and relaxed.

looking backward

This exercise is very simple in its execution but very profound in its effects.

1 Stand upright with your chest pushed out and your stomach pulled in. Let your hands hang at your sides, with your palms lightly touching your body.

2 Look straight ahead into the far distance and breathe in.

3 While exhaling, slowly turn your head clockwise as far as possible, as if you were trying to look at something directly behind you. Your feet should continue to face forward (see illustration).

4 Slowly return to the starting position and inhale deeply.

5 Repeat the exercise, turning your head counterclockwise. You may repeat the exercise 9 times in each direction. Only turn your head as far around as is comfortable. As you practice this exercise more, your flexibility will increase naturally, enabling you to turn further.

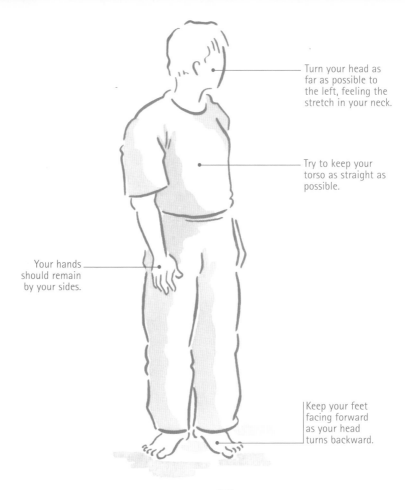

Turn your head as far as possible to the left, feeling the stretch in your neck.

Try to keep your torso as straight as possible.

Your hands should remain by your sides.

Keep your feet facing forward as your head turns backward.

looking backward

The more advanced form of the exercise is as follows:

❶ Stand with your legs together and your back straight. Let your arms hang down with your palms lightly touching your sides; look straight ahead.

❷ Take a step to the left and assume the Horse Riding Stance.

❸ Clench both hands into fists. Raise your left fist so that it is close to but not touching your abdomen. Raise your right fist to chest level.

❹ Turn your upper body to the left. Unclench your fists and push up with your right hand so that it is above your head on the right side, with your palm facing up. At the same time, drop your left arm so that it is parallel to your left leg, palm facing downward (see illustration). Turn your head counter-clockwise to look behind you.

❺ Return to the Horse Riding Stance with your fists in front of you. Repeat on the other side. Repeat 9 times on each side.

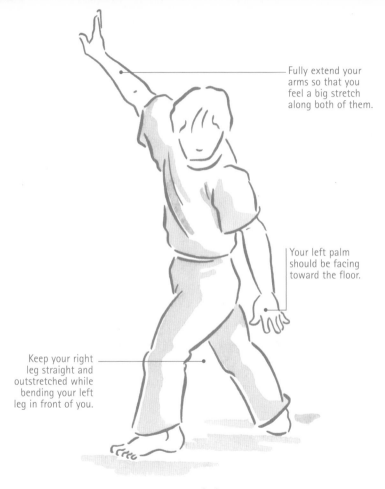

Fully extend your arms so that you feel a big stretch along both of them.

Your left palm should be facing toward the floor.

Keep your right leg straight and outstretched while bending your left leg in front of you.

looking backward

Looking Backward can be performed in a seated position.

❶ Sit comfortably with your back straight, either on a chair or cross-legged on the floor.

❷ Rest your hands on your knees with your palms down.

❸ Mentally visit every part of your body and allow each one to relax. For some muscles, it is easier to tense them first and then relax them.

❹ Roll your head in a half circle from left to right, looking backward as far as you can, and then from right to left (see illustration). Coordinate your breathing with your movements so that you inhale while lifting your head and exhale while lowering it.

❺ Repeat the exercise up to 9 times.

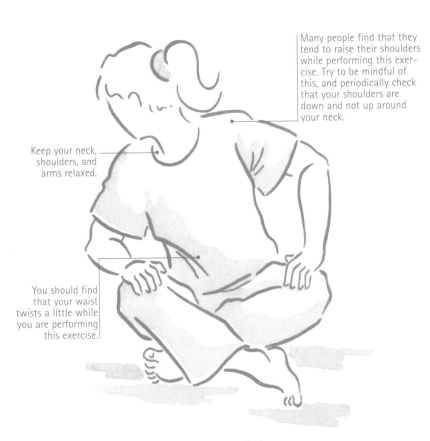

Many people find that they tend to raise their shoulders while performing this exercise. Try to be mindful of this, and periodically check that your shoulders are down and not up around your neck.

Keep your neck, shoulders, and arms relaxed.

You should find that your waist twists a little while you are performing this exercise.

the five elements

According to Chinese philosophy, the universe is manifested in the balance of opposite principles: yin and yang (see page 186). These principles work through the mechanism of Wu-Hsing—the Five Elements, or Five Material Agents. The theory of the Five Elements runs through all Chinese philosophy; it is one of the pillars of Chinese medicine, and part of the framework of various martial arts. The Five Elements are represented in nature by wood, fire, earth, metal, and water. Each has particular properties and is associated with certain seasons, colors, parts of the body, emotions, and phenomena, including politics and culture.

The early Taoists thought of each body organ as a field of intelligence, and they attributed to each one a positive and a negative emotion or energy. Each major organ is also associated with one of the Five Elements. For example, the liver is associated with the element wood; it has the positive emotion or energy of kindness and the negative emotion or energy of anger. The heart is associated with fire and has the positive energy of joy and the negative energy of hatred. In this way, each of us is connected to the Five Elements both emotionally and physically.

A chart of the elements and their associated properties is shown on the following pages.

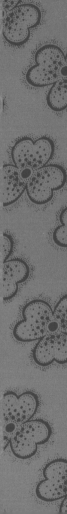

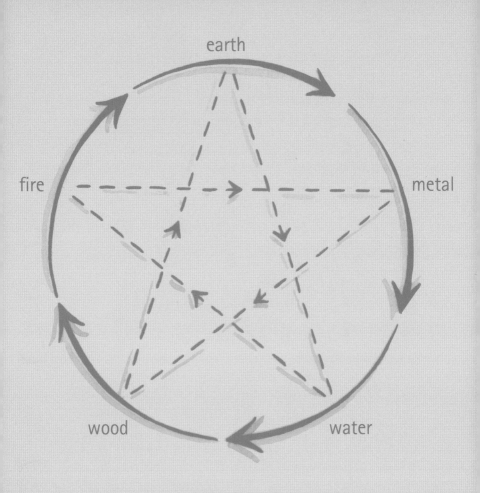

the five elements and their associated properties

The Five Elements generate and defeat each other in cycles (see page 77). They can be arranged in the order in which they produce each other: Wood produces fire, fire gives rise to earth, earth generates metal, metal engenders water, and water produces wood. Alternatively, they can be arranged in the order in which they destroy each other: Fire is quenched by water, water is conquered by earth, earth is defeated by wood, wood is subjugated by metal, and metal is liquidated by fire.

These cycles can be used to explain all change in the universe— including, of course, changes in the body. So if you have a disease of the liver, which is associated with the element wood, it is because wood is being defeated by the element metal. To cure the disease, you would need to use the energy of the element fire, because fire overcomes metal.

element	wood	fire	earth	metal	water
yin organ	liver	heart	spleen	lungs	kidneys
yang organ	gallbladder	small intestine	stomach	large intestine	bladder
color	green	red	yellow	white	black
direction	east	south	center	west	north
climate	wind	heat	humidity	dry	cold
season	spring	summer	late summer	fall	winter
beneficial emotion/energy	kindness	joy	groundedness	moral courage	courage
pathological emotion/energy	anger	hatred	worry	sorrow	fear
human sound	shouting	laughter	talking	weeping	groaning
sense organ	eyes	tongue	lips	nose	ears

what is meditation?

Meditation is a term with which everyone in the West is now familiar, though it has come to mean different things for different people. For some, it brings forth images of Buddhist monks living in monasteries shut away from society, sitting in strange postures for hours on end. You may feel that such a practice is out of reach for an "ordinary" person and so cannot benefit you. Fortunately, this is not the case. Meditation can be practiced in a wide range of places and contexts, and there are many different techniques that make the practice accessible to all.

But what exactly is meditation? One important component of all forms of meditation is concentration—you might say that meditation starts with concentration. Concentration is the capacity to hold your attention on one thing for an extended period of time. Some meditation techniques require you to hold your attention on only one object of concentration; others specify a range of targets until only one remains, and then even that is let go.

Meditation is also more than concentration: It involves selecting an object and then maintaining a flow of awareness toward that object. As you meditate on an object, you become increasingly aware of its true or essential nature. This may sound quite abstract, but it is actually a natural outcome of the **process of meditation**.

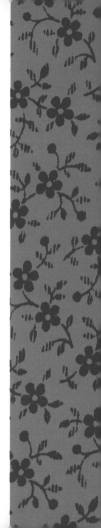

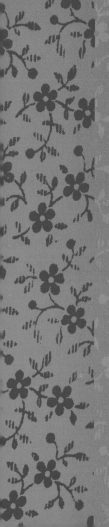

Details of the particular place and benefits of meditation in qigong practice are discussed later (see page 100). For now, here is an introduction to an enjoyable form of meditation that you can begin practicing immediately.

meditating in nature

Meditating in nature is a simple and rewarding exercise that can also be very exhilarating. On a day when the weather is good (not too extreme), choose a beautiful location where all five elements, wood, fire, earth, metal, and water, are present. Wood can be represented by trees, and fire by the sun. Earth can be represented by the ground, including rocks and mountains. Metal tends to be hidden—for example, as metal ores found underground. Anywhere that you are near earth, you are also likely to be near metal. Water can be represented by rivers, streams, and lakes. If you live in the city, you may find a suitable location in a local park, where features such as ponds and rock gardens enable you to be in touch with all the elements. Bring a cushion or blanket to sit on as you meditate.

If you want to focus on a single element, there are guided meditations throughout this book. The first is on water.

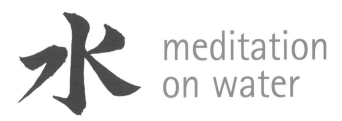 # meditation on water

Water is a nourishing, nurturing element, essential for life. Indeed, all forms of life on earth originally developed from water, and about two thirds of the human body itself is made up of water. We are even surrounded by water before birth, in the mother's womb.

Water can be purifying as well as nourishing, and if you harness the energies of water through meditation, it can have a deep cleansing effect on both your body and your mind.

The Meditation on Water can be especially beneficial if you have problems with your kidneys, bladder, or urinary or reproductive systems. People who suffer from fearfulness and need courage will also greatly benefit from this meditation.

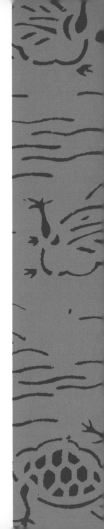

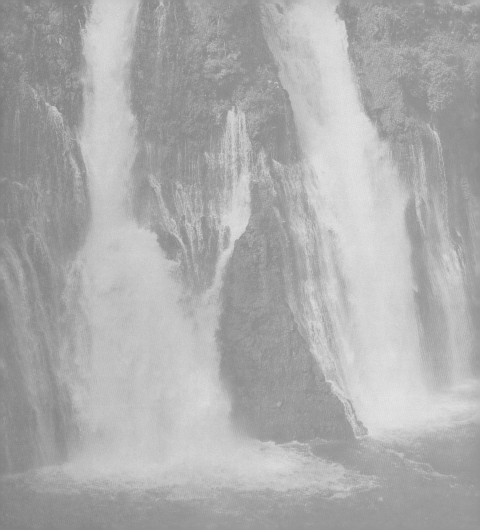

❶ This meditation may be performed indoors or outdoors. Meditating outdoors by a stream, lake, or other body of water is preferable. If you are indoors, turn on a tap a little so that you can hear the trickle of water. If it's raining, open a window and meditate near it. Alternatively, you could use a recording of environmental sounds as an object of concentration.

❷ Close your eyes. This will draw your senses inward and make you more perceptive of the environment around you.

❸ Make sure you are sitting comfortably with a straight back. Systematically relax your entire body, one part at a time, from the toes upward.

❹ Now listen to the sounds of the water. Feel it trickling, splashing, gurgling, or flowing serenely,

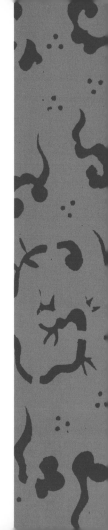

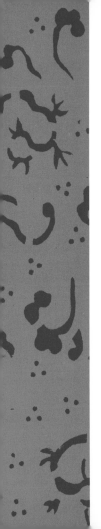

as appropriate. If thoughts come into your mind, gently let them go and bring your attention back to the sound of the water.

❺ If you are near a body of water but cannot hear it, breathe the water's energy toward you until you feel yourself immersed in it, then exhale the energy back into the body of water. Repeat 9 times, increasing in multiples of 9 up to 36 times as you become more advanced.

❻ After a few minutes, you will find your mind calmer and quieter. Enjoy this state for a few minutes more.

❼ When you are ready, gently bring yourself out of the meditative state. Rub your hands together, then rub your eyes and tap your body from your head down to your toes.

month5

Heaven lasts long, and Earth abides. What is the
secret of their durability?
Is it not because they do not live for
themselves, that they live for so long?
Therefore, the Sage wants to remain behind,
But he finds himself at the head of others;
Reckons himself out, but finds himself safe and
secure.
Is it not because he is selfless
That his Self is realized?

from the *Tao Te Ching*

contents:

Opening the treasure chest of qigong enhances your ability to draw energy from nature.

The fifth month is a month in which it is possible to observe how different organisms grow at different rates. Some plants are in full bloom, while others are still spreading roots beneath the soil, getting ready for their own moments in the sun. Similarly, in this month you will learn that anyone can practice and enjoy the benefits of qigong at his or her own pace. Whether you are young or old, male or female, you will certainly find mental, physical, and spiritual benefits from regular practice.

The Ba Duan Jin exercise Looking for Hidden Treasure is one of the most powerful exercises in the sequence. It strengthens your legs, tones your thighs and buttocks, and improves circulation to your feet. It also firms your waist, makes your lower back very supple, and improves the health

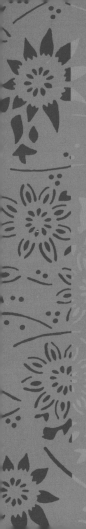

of the kidneys and pelvic region. But the greatest benefit by far is its soothing effect on the heart. This derives from the middle stage of the routine, when your torso is parallel to the floor. This position helps you to regain one advantage that was lost to humans when we began to walk upright—in many quadrupedal animals, the heart pumps blood more or less parallel to the ground, whereas in humans, it must pump vertically against gravity.

By this point in your qigong year, you should also have a greater understanding of meditation and its importance in qigong, and, as you learn to fully relax and allow all extraneous thoughts to disappear from your head, you will start to experience even greater benefits to your general health and well-being.

The second of the Meditations on the Elements, this time on wood, is particularly beneficial if you have liver problems or often find yourself getting angry or frustrated. However, the liver is such an important organ in the body that this meditation is extremely beneficial to anyone, regardless of their physical and mental health.

looking for hidden treasure

This exercise should be done in a continuous, mindful flow.
It is important that you progress into this exercise gradually
—do not bend your knees more than is comfortable. As your
leg muscles become stronger through practice, you will
comfortably be able to bend your knees through nearly 90
degrees without even thinking about it. Such natural
progress is part of the beauty of regular practice.

❶ Stand with your feet shoulder-width apart and your feet
pointing forward. Lower your torso by bending your knees
at approximately 45 degrees.

❷ Place your hands on your thighs (see illustration). This
position is similar to the Horse Riding Stance.

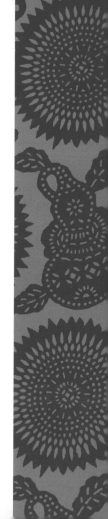

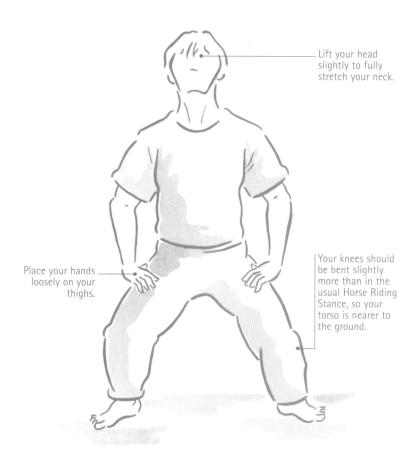

Lift your head slightly to fully stretch your neck.

Place your hands loosely on your thighs.

Your knees should be bent slightly more than in the usual Horse Riding Stance, so your torso is nearer to the ground.

[91]

❸ Bend forward from the waist until your torso is almost horizontal (see illustration).

❹ Raise your torso upward toward the right with a twisting motion so that you end up facing right, with your buttocks pointing to the left. Your left arm will naturally straighten. Keep your right arm bent (see illustration). It is important that you are able to support your legs in this bent position throughout these movements, so do not try to bend your legs beyond the point of comfort.

❺ Face forward. Now twist and turn your torso upward to the left without straightening your knees, allowing your right arm to straighten while your left arm remains bent.

❻ Repeat the exercise 9 times on each side.

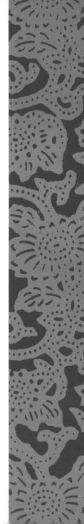

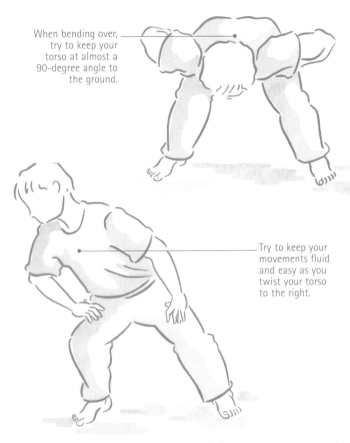

When bending over, try to keep your torso at almost a 90-degree angle to the ground.

Try to keep your movements fluid and easy as you twist your torso to the right.

looking for hidden treasure

A more advanced form of the exercise is as follows:

1 Stand with your feet shoulder-width apart, with your legs and back straight. Look straight ahead.

2 Place your hands in front of your waist with your palms facing upward. Your fingertips should be pointing toward each other but not touching.

3 Bend forward at the waist. Try to keep your back straight.

4 Drop your arms down toward your toes.

5 Turn your head to the left and twist your buttocks to the right (see illustration).

6 Smoothly raise your torso to an upright position. Your hands should be at waist level and your palms facing upward.

7 Repeat on the other side, turning your head to the right and your buttocks to the left. Repeat 9 times on each side.

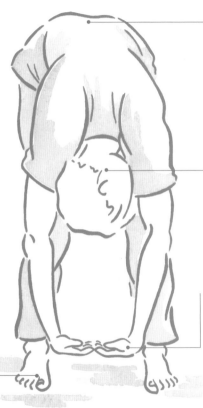

Thrust your buttocks out sideways to the right, feeling the stretch down your left leg.

At the same time, make sure your head is facing toward the left, which creates a stretch down the right side.

Try to get your hands as near to the floor as possible, keeping your back straight to maximize the stretch.

Your feet should still be pointing straight ahead.

looking for hidden treasure

The seated version of Looking for Hidden Treasure delivers similar health benefits to the standing versions.

❶ Sit comfortably on a firm chair with your back straight. Keep your knees together with both feet firmly on the floor.

❷ Bend forward from your waist, keeping your movements as smooth as possible. Try to touch the floor.

❸ While keeping your knees down, your arms stretched, and your back straight, try to get your forehead down as close as possible to your knees (see illustration).

❹ Sit up and repeat a total of 9 times.

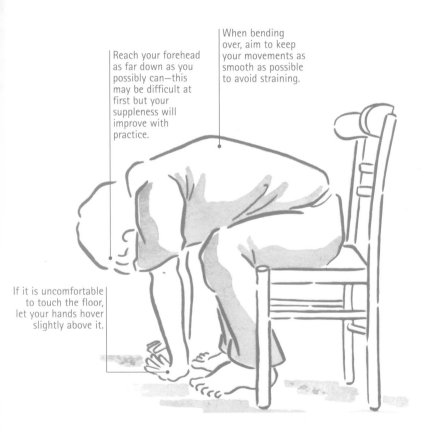

Reach your forehead as far down as you possibly can—this may be difficult at first but your suppleness will improve with practice.

When bending over, aim to keep your movements as smooth as possible to avoid straining.

If it is uncomfortable to touch the floor, let your hands hover slightly above it.

five elements, three cycles

The Five Elements that are the mechanism for all change in the universe are related to each other through three cycles. There are two schools of thought regarding how the ancient Chinese developed knowledge of the cycles; one school says that they perceived this knowledge through meditation, while the other maintains that they simply observed nature closely. Perhaps a combination of the two yielded the theory.

One cycle elucidated by the ancients is as follows: Water nourishes plants and hence generates wood. Wood burns, giving rise to fire. When matter burns, ashes remain, so fire generates earth. Metals lie in the earth and have to be mined, so earth can be said to generate metal. Water vapor condenses on metal to give rise to water, so metal generates water. This cycle is called the constructive or creative cycle. Each element is the mother of the element it generates and the son of the element that generated it. For example, fire is the son of wood and the mother of earth.

The destructive cycle describes how the elements inhibit, control, or destroy each other. Wood destroys earth as plants deplete the soil of nutrients. Metal destroys wood as an axe can split a log. Fire melts metal; water extinguishes fire. Earth overcomes water, since it can block the flow of rivers and ocean waves.

The creative and destructive cycles (shown in the diagram below) balance each other and promote normal development. However, there is a third cycle (not shown), called the counteracting cycle, that arises when one element is too weak to overcome another element as it normally should. As a result, nature becomes temporarily out of balance. For example, water usually overcomes fire. If a fire rages too fiercely, though, it can vaporize the water rather than the water extinguishing the fire. In this way, water is conquered by fire.

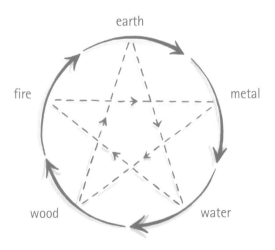

meditation and qigong

In qigong meditation, the focus is on qi—sensing qi, feeling it travel around your body, and moving it in prescribed ways so that your entire body is activated and its energies are harmonized. This leaves your mind balanced and calm and your body healthy and strong. Other meditations have different aims—for example, Buddhist meditation is concerned with enlightenment; other techniques emphasize relaxation.

Qigong masters strongly recommend that you spend some time meditating after practicing qigong exercises. This will further calm your mind, relax your body, and renew your energy levels. Meditation allows negative, pathological energy to leave your body so that you can be recharged by the universal life force. During meditation, as well as during qigong routines, you may feel qi moving around your body. The movement of qi may feel like tingling, tickling, heat, or heaviness; you may also sense the movement visually as changing colors.

Good meditative practice clears your meridians (the energetic pathways in your body along which qi travels) of obstructions. If you are able to reach a deep level of meditation, you will be able to heal not only yourself but others, too. For centuries, Chinese and Indian yogis have used meditation to heal.

letting thoughts go

While meditating, try to let go of yourself and your thoughts. Ideally, you need to forget yourself completely. It is not easy to let go of your conscious mind, but it does become easier with practice. You may find that you have good days, when your mind easily frees itself of thoughts, and some days that are not quite so good. As your practice intensifies, you will find that the proportion of good days increases.

If your mind starts racing, thinking about tasks that need to be accomplished or ways to solve a particular problem, try to talk deliberately to your mind. Try telling it to be quiet for the moment and that you will allow it time to work out whatever problems plague it after you have finished meditating. After meditating, your mind will be more relaxed and tranquil and better able to focus on its tasks.

If you have a problem and are unsure about what action to take, it often helps to spend a few minutes thinking about it, trying to get as clear a picture of it as possible, before you begin meditating. Then let the picture disappear from your mind and begin meditating. After meditating, you will most likely find that you have an even clearer picture of the problem and that a solution is therefore more apparent.

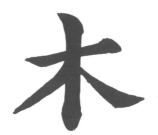 # meditation on wood

According to the theory of the Five Elements, wood is associated with the liver. The related beneficial energy is kindness, while the harmful or pathological energy is anger. If you suffer from liver problems or become angry quickly, this meditation is particularly suited to you.

When you practice the Meditation on Wood, you gain a deeper understanding of trees as amazing organisms. They remain in the same place all year round, withstanding the heat of summer and the cold of winter. They send their roots deep into the soil and draw life-giving water and minerals from its depths. Their roots also anchor them and make them almost immovable. Using the energy of the sun, they convert water and carbon dioxide into food. This is what the practitioner of qigong is ultimately trying to emulate.

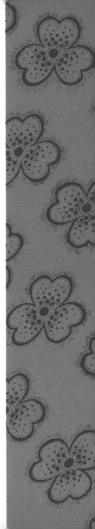

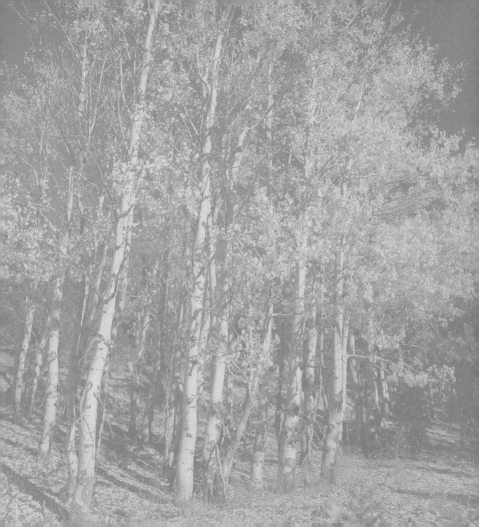

❶ A suitable location for this meditation is at the base of a large tree. Find a tree that particularly attracts your attention—you will find that this is the tree that has the right energetic relationship to you. As you approach the tree, mentally greet it. Ask it to share its tremendous healing energy with you and to assist you in removing any pathological or negative energy from your body. You may want to gently bow to the tree.

❷ Spread a blanket on the ground underneath the tree. Sit down on it, cross-legged, making sure that you are feeling comfortable and relaxed. Your back should be as straight as possible—visualizing a thread that connects the top of your head to the sky may help you keep your spine straight and tall. Tucking in your chin slightly will further align your back.

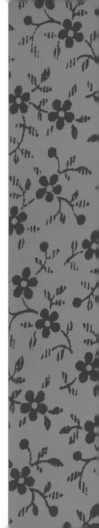

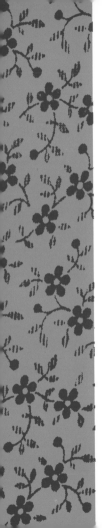

❸ Close your eyes to draw your senses inward and become more perceptive of the environment around you.

❹ Systematically relax your entire body, starting with your feet. To do this, bring your attention to your feet and instruct them to relax. Next, bring your attention to your lower legs and tell them to relax. Gradually move up the body, relaxing your upper legs, hips, pelvis, abdomen and chest. Then move on to your arms and your head. After a while, your whole body should feel loose and relaxed.

❺ Now try to feel that you are one with nature. One way to do this is to reflect on the similarities between your environment and your body—the water element found in rivers and streams is equivalent to your blood, wood and trees correspond to your bones, the sky corresponds to the vast nature of your mind, and the clouds correspond to your thoughts, which come and go. Do this for at least 10 minutes.

❻ Now become aware of the sounds around you—the rustling of leaves, the creaking of the branches. Start by focusing on the sound that seems most prominent, then explore successively quieter sounds one by one.

❼ By now you will be feeling very peaceful and deeply relaxed; you will also sense that you are part of the wonderful movement of energy that is nature.

❽ As you breathe, visualize that you are exchanging energy with the tree. As you inhale, imagine that you are drawing in healing energy

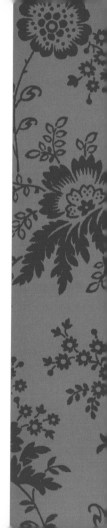

from the tree; as you exhale, imagine that the tree is drawing away your pathological or negative energy. The tree channels this energy away from you into the earth, via its roots. You will soon become aware that this is a very real process. At this point in the meditation, you may feel a mild tingling sensation similar to an electric current as a flow of energy moves between you and the tree with each inhalation and exhalation.

❾ Perform 36 of these breath cycles, and then sit still, keeping your mind free from thought. If any thoughts come, let them go. Your mind should resemble a sky without clouds.

❿ When you are ready, gently bring yourself out of the meditative state. Rub your hands together, then rub your eyes and, forming your hand into a fist, tap your body all over.

month6

Thirty spokes converge upon a single hub;
It is on the hole in the center that the use of
   the cart hinges.
We make a vessel from a lump of clay;
It is the empty space within the vessel that
   makes it useful.
We make doors and windows for a room;
But it is these empty spaces that make the
   room liveable.
Thus, while the tangible has advantages,
It is the intangible that makes it useful.

from the *Tao Te Ching*

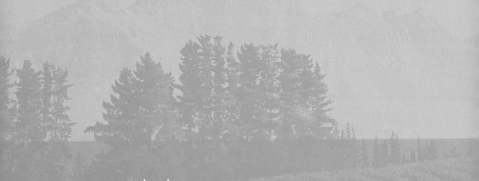

contents:

See the young shoots growing from the seeds of your practice.

If you are a gardener and have sown seeds, you know that it takes a while to see the fruits of your labor. Some seeds you planted in early spring may not yet have begun to sprout. Similarly, having started to practice qigong, you may wonder how long it will take to see results. This period varies from individual to individual, but the ancients did leave some general guidelines: In the first 100 days, you should see some definite signs of improvement. After 1000 days of dedicated practice, results will be self-evident. It is essential to practice on a regular basis—a few minutes every day will bear fruit quicker than practicing in fits and starts.

The Ba Duan Jin exercise for this month is called Touching the Earth. In physical terms, this exercise strengthens the back and waist muscles through forward

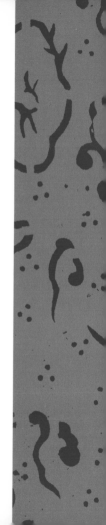

and backward stretching. The exercise has profound systemic benefits, especially for the kidneys. If you find yourself frequently getting up at night to urinate, if you suffer from pain in the lower back, or if you have bladder or prostate problems, then this exercise can be especially helpful for you. In addition, traditional Chinese medicine believes that the kidneys are related to the reproductive organs, so this exercise can help ease painful periods and PMS. The sitting variation of this exercise is good for keeping the shoulders, arms, and elbows supple, thus preventing ailments in those areas. It also increases circulation and helps open up the chest.

In this month there is a discussion on the best direction to face while practicing qigong. Each point of the compass is associated with a different element, so by facing in one direction you can harness the energy of that direction's element to help heal a specific ailment.

The third Meditation on the Elements, the Meditation on Earth, is very beneficial if you have problems with your digestive system; it will also help you relax.

touching the earth

This exercise gives you an opportunity to become grounded and to communicate with the earth itself, as well as encouraging the flow of qi in the lower back, hips, and legs.

❶ Stand upright with your feet and legs together, your back and knees straight, and your arms hanging at your sides with your palms facing inward. Look straight ahead.

❷ Breathe in deeply as you raise your arms so that your hands draw an arc in front of you. Continue to raise your arms until they are vertically extended above your head. Bend backward slightly to emphasize the stretch.

❸ As you exhale, bring your arms back down in front of you and bend from your waist until your hands touch the floor (see illustration).

❹ Repeat the exercise 9 times in total.

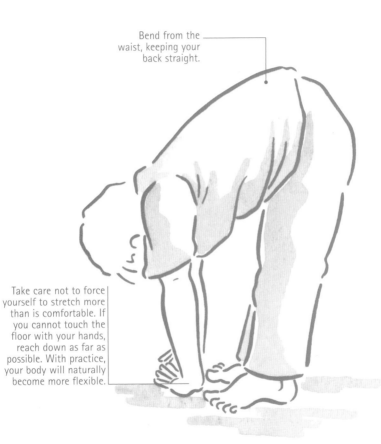

Bend from the waist, keeping your back straight.

Take care not to force yourself to stretch more than is comfortable. If you cannot touch the floor with your hands, reach down as far as possible. With practice, your body will naturally become more flexible.

touching the earth

Once you have mastered the basic form, you may proceed
to the advanced form.

❶ Stand upright with your feet and legs together, your
back and knees straight, and your arms hanging at your
sides with your palms facing inward. Look straight ahead.

❷ Without bending either leg at the knee, raise your left
leg from the hip so that it points straight out in front of
you and is parallel to the ground.

❸ Hold the toes of your left foot with both hands and
look straight ahead (see illustration).

❹ Let go of your left foot and allow your leg to return to
the ground.

❺ Return to the starting position and repeat the exercise
with your right leg.

❻ You may repeat the exercise up to 9 times on each side.

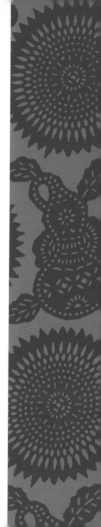

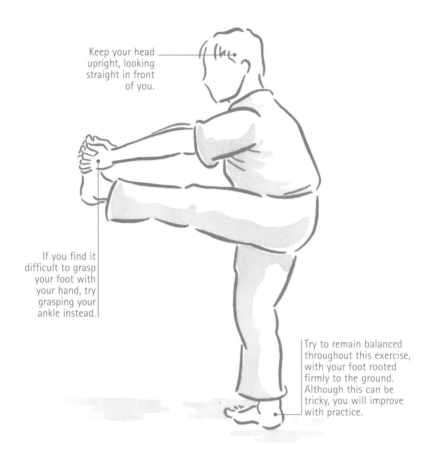

Keep your head upright, looking straight in front of you.

If you find it difficult to grasp your foot with your hand, try grasping your ankle instead.

Try to remain balanced throughout this exercise, with your foot rooted firmly to the ground. Although this can be tricky, you will improve with practice.

touching the earth

The seated form of Touching the Earth involves wheeling your arms around in front of you.

❶ Sit on the floor in a comfortable position with your back straight.

❷ Extend your legs out in front of you. Try to keep your knees straight and together.

❸ Extend both arms straight in front of you. Make a fist with both hands. Your palms should be facing each other but not touching (see illustration).

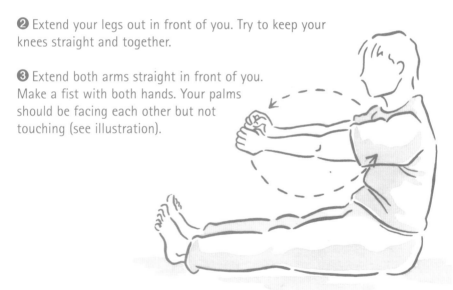

❹ Draw vertical circles in front of you with your fists, as if you were turning the pedals of a bicycle (your hands will move in opposition to each other; see illustration). Draw 9 complete circles clockwise followed by 9 circles counterclockwise. Keep your upper body loose so that your head and shoulders sway in rhythm to your arms.

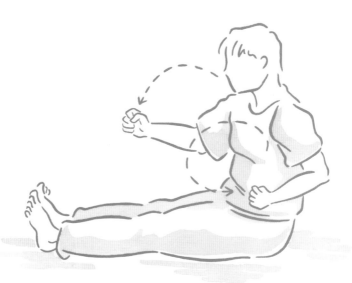

elements, emotions, and ailments

Last month you discovered how you are connected to the Five Elements, both physically and emotionally. If you look at the table featured on page 79, you will see that each element has certain parts of the body associated with it. In traditional Chinese medicine, the Theory of the Five Elements is used for diagnosis and treatment of diseases. Each element finds release for its negative energy. For example, if you suffer from kidney problems, you probably also have back problems, particularly lower back problems. Kidney problems are also associated with a lack of energy and feeling tired, insecure, and frightened. This may result in a lot of moaning and groaning. By complaining to others, you release negative energy from your kidneys.

Similarly, if you have liver problems, you tend to be angry or frustrated. You may find release for negative energy by shouting. If you have heart problems, hatred may be a vehicle for you to release the negative energy of your heart. If you suffer from stomach or digestive problems, you may use talking as a way of releasing negative energy. And if you have a lung disorder, you may tend to feel sad or depressed. In this case, crying may help release negative lung energy.

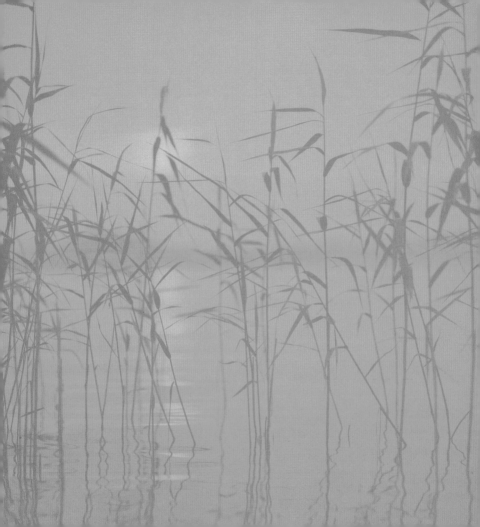

directions, emotions, and ailments

Each of the Five Elements has an associated direction. These directions relate to different internal organs. You can enhance your qigong practice by facing in the direction appropriate to your ailment. For instance, if you have a problem with your kidneys or reproductive organs, face north. Face south if you have a problem with your heart or circulatory system. Face east if you have a liver or gallbladder disorder. If you have a a lung disorder, face west. If you have a problem with your stomach, spleen, or pancreas, you can face whichever direction you like, because these organs are associated with the center.

However, if you have an excess of the pathological energy or emotion associated with a particular organ, you should face the opposite direction. Bear in mind that an excess is due to the yang principle; a weakness or deficiency is due to the yin principle. Imbalances between yin and yang cause health problems, so the goal is to bring these two energies into a state of equilibrium. For example, if you are quick to anger, then you have too much yang energy in your liver. In this case, when doing your qigong practice, you should face the direction opposite that of the liver— west. If you suffer from hatred, cruelty, or excessive joy, you should face

north. Face south if you suffer from fear, east if you suffer from sadness, and west if you suffer from anger or frustration. If you suffer from worry or anxiety, you can face any direction, because these emotions are associated with the center.

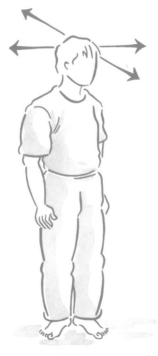

meditation and the energies in nature

Stress is now a major health issue in our society, partly due to our hectic modern lifestyles, but also because our relationship with nature has been partially severed through lack of contact—we walk on concrete, drink cola, eat highly processed foods, and drive everywhere. Meditation can help to calm the mind, relieving the buildup of the daily stresses that can lead to disease. By focusing on the five elements (see page 76–79), you can reestablish your connection with nature and allow it to nurture you.

Each element of nature is also represented in the body. When you focus on an element in meditation, you become sensitive to it, attuning yourself to its vibrational energies. You then learn to absorb its qi. By balancing the qi of each element in your body, you develop harmony in body, mind, and emotions. As you increase your efficiency at drawing in the qi of each element, you can learn to balance the elemental forces in your body (see page 78) by drawing in the energies that are weak in your body, or by focusing on those that overcome an element that is strong.

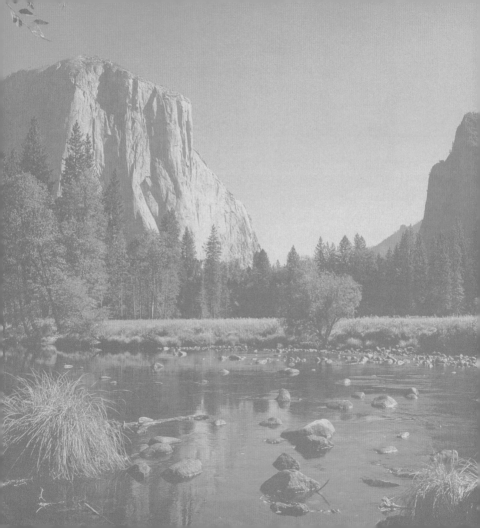

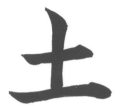

meditation on earth

The earth element, which is associated with the digestive system, is particularly significant for many people, because our diet and lifestyle can create digestive disorders. Meditating on the earth element can help prevent and alleviate these problems.

Many cultures have realized the importance of the earth as a positive force. Clay is widely used as a healing tool. People enjoy working with clay, and it is frequently used in therapy. In aboriginal cultures, sick people are laid in the earth; in parts of the Middle East, mud baths are renowned for their health-giving properties; and in the West, many people use mudpacks to cleanse the skin. Thus, the importance of the earth element is not confined solely to qigong theory and Chinese culture.

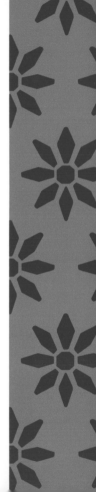

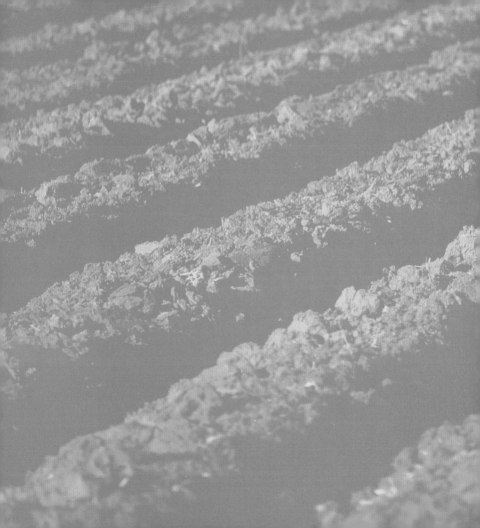

Meditation on earth

❶ This meditation is best done outdoors, while sitting or standing on the earth, establishing direct contact with its energies. If this isn't possible for you, then make sure that your feet are touching the ground throughout the meditation. This is easy if you are standing; but if you choose to sit down, you could sit with your knees up and the soles of your feet on the floor. With time, you will be able to feel the vibrational energy of the earth. Whether you are sitting or standing, be sure to keep your back as straight as possible.

❷ Tell each part of your body to relax in turn, starting with the feet and working your way up.

❸ Try to become sensitive to the earth's energy. Feel the ground beneath you; feel at one with it. If it helps, visualize yourself surrounded by earth.

❹ Feel the earth's healing energy entering and filling your body and energizing your abdomen. Breathe in this energy. As you breathe out, expel all the negative energy in your body into the depths of the earth. Repeat this breathing exercise in cycles of 9, building up to a total of 36 breathing cycles.

❺ Now take the time to spend a few minutes free of thoughts. Sit quietly and simply enjoy the earth around you. If any thoughts do come into your mind, quickly let them go and bring your mind back to your breathing.

❻ When you are ready to come out of the meditation, rub your hands together and gently brush down your entire body. You should feel relaxed and refreshed and ready to enjoy the rest of your day.

fall

consolidation

By this point in the qigong year, your body will be more balanced and working as a harmonious unit, your energy levels will have increased, and your health will have improved. Friends may have begun to notice a change in you. However, it is important not to become complacent. Just as animals prepare for the winter months, so must you continue to practice diligently, so that you continue to grow and come to new realizations that will benefit your life in numerous ways. Fall is also the time when the trees shed their leaves—you too may find yourself casting off unwanted habits which previously seemed so difficult to break.

month 7
month 8
month 9

month 7

The highest type of ruler is one of whose
    existence the people are barely aware.
Next comes one whom they love and praise.
Next comes one whom they fear.
Next comes one whom they despise and defy.
When you are lacking in faith, others will be
    unfaithful to you.
The Sage is self-effacing and scanty of words.
When his task is accomplished and things have
    been completed,
All the people say, "We ourselves have achieved it!"

from the *Tao Te Ching*

contents:

Let your qigong practice grow steadily—don't let it be like a lightning flash in a summer storm.

The seventh month is a time of consolidating the stores of our harvest. By this point in your qigong year, you will be acquiring knowledge and expertise at a steady and constant rate. As with most exercise routines, a good depth of knowledge and true efficiency can really be achieved only by regular and diligent practice. Moreover, working at a comfortable pace and not rushing can enable you to build up your repository of qigong knowledge, which in turn enables you to reap the full benefits of qigong. In this month, the importance of practice is examined.

Regular practice of the seventh exercise in the Ba Duan Jin sequence, Reaching Out to Nature, can have dramatic effects on your concentration because of the rhythmic nature of the movements. The exercise also builds up physical energy and strength, especially in the arms and shoulders, and, in the standing variations, in the legs and buttocks. It also has a great revitalizing effect on inner organs such as the liver and the heart. This exercise—which can sometimes be known as Punching with Angry Eyes because of an ancient tradition of glaring angrily while carrying out the movements—is also very beneficial to your mental health, in that it helps to get rid of inner tension and frustration and brings you back to a balanced state of mind.

The fourth of the Meditations on the Elements, the Meditation on Fire, will help you to stay connected to the warmth associated with this month. This meditation is particularly beneficial if you suffer from heart, respiratory, or circulatory problems, such as cold hands and feet. It's also helpful to meditate on fire if you tend to feel a lot of envy or hatred—this meditation can bring more joy into your life.

reaching out to nature

As with any qigong exercise, try to follow the movements with your mind or, alternatively, keep your mind on your breathing or free from thought. It's difficult to still the mind, so don't expect that you will be able to do so immediately. Success comes with concentration and plenty of practice.

❶ Stand with your feet shoulder-width apart, bend your knees, look straight ahead, and assume the Horse Riding Stance.

❷ Make fists with both hands and raise them to just above your hips, with the palms facing upward and your elbows pointing directly backward (see illustration).

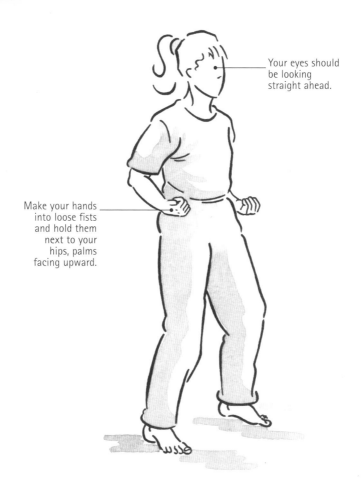

Your eyes should be looking straight ahead.

Make your hands into loose fists and hold them next to your hips, palms facing upward.

❸ Stretch your left fist straight out in front of you so that your knuckles point away from your body and your palm faces down (see illustration).

❹ Inhale deeply. As you exhale through your mouth, extend your right arm so that its position mirrors that of your left arm. At the same time, bring your left fist to your left hip, palm facing upward. As your arm becomes fully extended, stare into the distance, tense your entire arm, and then relax it.

❺ Repeat these movements, alternately extending and retracting your arms. You will need to rotate your arms toward the end of each movement so that the palm of the extended arm faces up and that of the retracted arm faces down. You can also add a small thrusting or punching motion as your arm reaches its full extension.

❻ After 9 repetitions on each side, drop both arms to your sides and raise yourself from the Horse Riding Stance. With your body upright and your legs together, look straight ahead.

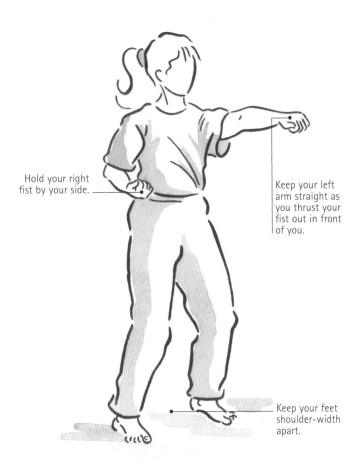

Hold your right fist by your side.

Keep your left arm straight as you thrust your fist out in front of you.

Keep your feet shoulder-width apart.

reaching out to nature

A more advanced form of the exercise is as follows:

1 Stand with your back straight and your legs together. Let your arms hang down with your palms lightly touching your sides. Look straight ahead.

2 Take a step to the left. Lower yourself into the Horse Riding Stance.

3 Make fists with both hands and bring each fist to just above the corresponding hip, with your palms facing up and your elbows pointing directly back.

4 Staring ahead, hold this position for as long as is comfortable (up to a few minutes). With more practice, you will be able to hold this position longer.

5 Slowly rise from the Horse Riding Stance and return to the starting position.

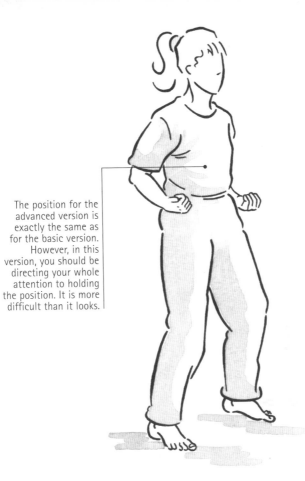

The position for the advanced version is exactly the same as for the basic version. However, in this version, you should be directing your whole attention to holding the position. It is more difficult than it looks.

reaching out to nature

A form of this exercise can also be done while seated:

❶ Sit comfortably with your back straight, either on the ground or in a straight-backed chair.

❷ Clench your hands into fists. Bring both fists to touch the sides of your body at waist level, palms facing up. Your elbows should be bent and pointing back.

❸ Thrust your right fist forward (see illustration). Rotate your arm so that your palm faces down when your arm is fully extended. Bring your right fist back to your waist, rotating it so your palm faces up, while thrusting your left fist forward as you did with your right fist.

❹ Repeat the exercise, thrusting your fists to the sides rather than to the front.

❺ Repeat again, this time thrusting your fists across your body so that your right fist goes to the left and your left fist goes to the right. Repeat each variation 9 times.

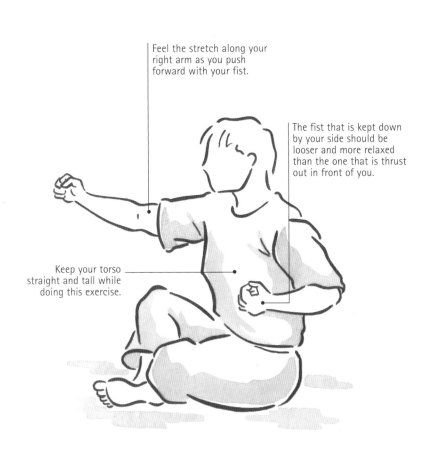

Feel the stretch along your right arm as you push forward with your fist.

The fist that is kept down by your side should be looser and more relaxed than the one that is thrust out in front of you.

Keep your torso straight and tall while doing this exercise.

the importance of practice

A session of qigong will certainly raise the level of qi in your body, contributing to your sense of well-being. But only with regular daily practice will you find you are able to maintain good health, or improve poor health. For maximum impact, you need to develop an adequate level of proficiency, and to do so, according to Taoist teachings, you must practice for 100 consecutive days. Self-discipline is the key to success at the start of your new routine, until it becomes part of your lifestyle. Focus on your goal—to live in health with peace of mind—and use this to compound your determination.

For success in your qigong practice, consider carefully how to incorporate it into your daily life. Having a regular routine means you are less likely to forget your practice or schedule other tasks for the same time period. The time of day that you set aside for practice is important. Choose a time when you are able to practice in a calm, relaxed state of mind, with no noise or interruptions. Given the pace of modern life, many people find it easier to develop a morning and evening routine. Exercise and meditate first thing in the morning to energize you for the day's challenges, and last thing at night to prepare yourself for a good night's sleep.

Short, regular, concentrated sessions are ideal for setting up a new routine, so begin with one or two 20-minute sessions each day. If there is more time available, extend your practice to 30 minutes or more. Should you find that you can spare only 5 to 10 minutes a day, then use it to practice qigong and meditation—you will still benefit. Daily practice is of utmost importance. It will build your proficiency, and you will soon notice signs of progress. Also, if you practice for 20 minutes in the morning and 20 minutes in the evening—regularly and with attention—you will increase the level of qi within your body and release blocked energy and tension as they build up in your body, before they become serious problems.

Performing qigong in a natural setting, especially one that you have a special feeling for, such as your own garden or a local park, is ideal, but in a daily routine for town and city dwellers, it sometimes isn't practical. Instead, try giving some attention to the space in your home in which you practice. It should be a peaceful and relaxing space rather than one filled with clutter, and should be away from noise or bustle. Clear a space especially for your practice if necessary. The clothing you choose is also important. Collect a small selection of loose-fitting T-shirts and baggy running pants, so you always have a store of clean clothes for your practice.

# meditation on fire

Fire is an ancient, primordial force. The sun, a fiery ball, is the prime source of energy on earth and sustains all life. It has also long been worshipped as a source of spiritual power. Humans learned to live successfully on earth when they harnessed the power of fire. As well as providing physical warmth and light, fire is seen as a vital energizing force within the body, the basis of all metabolic processes.

Harnessing the energies of fire through meditation is beneficial if you have heart, respiratory, or circulatory problems (such as cold hands or feet). It's also helpful if you tend to feel a lot of envy or hatred.

As you perform this routine, it is essential that you try not to visualize any smoke, since this may have detrimental effects on the meditation.

❶ You can meditate on fire indoors or outdoors. You don't literally need to be next to a fire to perform the meditation, but if you do have an open fire in your home, try meditating in front of it, or make a small campfire if you are meditating outdoors. Alternatively, you can meditate on a hot day so you can feel the sun's fiery heat.

❷ Sit upright with your back straight. Visualizing a thread connecting the top of your head with the sky will help to keep your spine aligned.

❸ Relax your entire body by telling each part to relax in turn, starting with the feet and working your way up to the head.

❹ Look deeply into the fire. If you are not actually sitting in front of a fire, imagine that you are surrounded by a ring of fire or facing an imposing mountain covered in flames. Look at the beautiful dance of the flames and feel their heat entering your body, warming it through and awakening its inner vitality.

❺ As you absorb the warmth of the fire, imagine that you are also absorbing its healthy energy, while your negative energy leaves your body and is quickly consumed by the flames.

❻ Stay in this meditative state for a few minutes. Try to let all your thoughts go. As in the other meditations, if your mind wanders, gently bring it back to the object of meditation—in this case, the fire.

❼ Slowly bring yourself out of the meditation, rub your hands together, and brush yourself down from head to toe.

month8

Heaviness is the root of lightness. Serenity is
the master of restlessness.
Therefore, the Sage, traveling all day, does not
part with the baggage-wagon.
Though there may be gorgeous sights to see, he
stays at ease in his own home.
Why should a lord of ten thousand chariots
Display his lightness to the world?
To be light is to be separated from one's root,
To be restless is to lose one's self-mastery.

From the *Tao Te Ching*

contents:

Let waves of energy wash over you like sand on the beach.

Month eight, the pinnacle of fall, is a time when shores feel the full force of the ocean's energy, brought on by hurricanes and storms at sea. This month, you will discover how to use your own waves of energy to unblock your body's meridians and improve health and vitality. Generating Waves of Energy, the last of the eight Ba Duan Jin exercises, includes an excellent sitting routine that relaxes and loosens the entire body.

The Meditation on metal is especially beneficial if you have respiratory problems.

By the time you have finished this chapter, you will have completed all eight of the Ba Duan Jin exercises at various levels. You should already have noticed dramatic changes in your suppleness, strength, and energy levels. Each of the Ba Duan Jin exercises works on a different part of the body and stimulates different organs. Many of the benefits come from the combination of movement and deep breathing. For maximum benefit, do the entire set of Ba Duan Jin exercises in sequence, but which variation of each exercise you choose is up to you. Regularly practicing all the Ba Duan Jin routines has the following general benefits:

- It strengthens the tendons, bones, and muscles.
- It improves circulation, especially to the extremities, ensuring that the vital organs remain well nourished.
- It enhances the immune system, providing greater resistance to colds and disease in general.
- It calms and balances the nervous system.

You have also probably felt some powerful effects from meditating on the Five Elements. These meditations reinforce the energy gained during the Qigong exercises. They bring both mind and body into balance. Once you have learned all the meditations, you may choose to follow one in particular that speaks to you, combined with the qigong exercises that you prefer.

generating waves of energy

This exercise is designed to open blocked meridians and improve the circulation of qi throughout your body. If you perform it properly, you will feel waves of energy course through your body, from your feet to your head. It is essential to relax completely during this exercise. Some people tend to tense up in order to avoid experiencing the full impact of the exercise. Although you may experience some unpleasant sensations if your body is full of toxins, such as a slight headache, this will soon dissipate as the beneficial effects of the exercise take hold. Regularly practicing Generating Waves of Energy improves blood flow to the internal organs, which helps detoxify them. In addition, your mind will feel clearer and your senses will be brighter and sharper.

❶ Stand with your feet shoulder-width apart. Let your arms hang loosely at your sides.

❷ Look straight ahead into the distance. Make sure your shoulders are relaxed, and empty your mind of all thoughts.

❸ After a few minutes, begin to rise up onto the balls of your feet (see illustration). When you are on your tiptoes, allow your body to sink back down onto your heels. With time, you will feel waves of energy traveling up to your head.

❹ Repeat the exercise a total of 9 times, and then take a short walk around the room to relax your body.

Try to keep the movement of rising onto the balls of your feet and sinking back onto your heels fluid and relaxed.

generating waves of energy

This exercise can be taken to two further levels.

trotting level

1 Stand with both feet slightly wider than shoulder-width apart. Let your arms hang loosely at your sides.

2 Lower your body into the Horse Riding Stance.

3 Raise your left hand to the middle of your chest and form a fist, as if you were holding some reins.

4 Bring your right hand to your side and slightly behind you. Form a fist with your right hand as if you were holding a whip (see illustration). At the same time, raise and drop your heels in rapid succession.

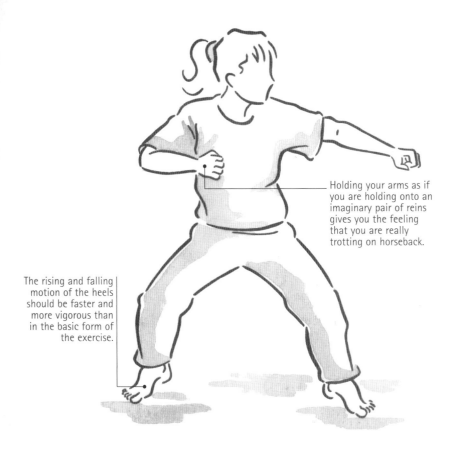

Holding your arms as if you are holding onto an imaginary pair of reins gives you the feeling that you are really trotting on horseback.

The rising and falling motion of the heels should be faster and more vigorous than in the basic form of the exercise.

[155]

generating waves of energy
galloping level

❶ Stand with both feet slightly wider than shoulder-width apart. Let your arms hang loosely at your sides.

❷ Lower your body into the Horse Riding Stance.

❸ Lean forward and stretch both arms in front of you, with your palms open (see illustration).

❹ Raise and drop your heels in rapid succession. While you are doing this, shake your whole body as if you were on a galloping horse.

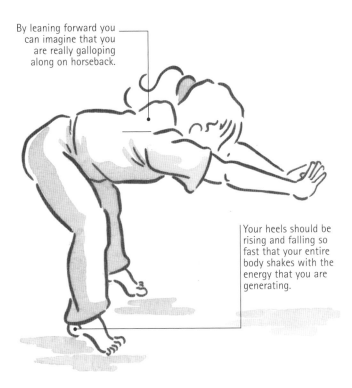

By leaning forward you can imagine that you are really galloping along on horseback.

Your heels should be rising and falling so fast that your entire body shakes with the energy that you are generating.

ba duan jin closing exercise

This exercise loosens and relaxes all muscles and nerves in the body, and it is an excellent closing exercise for the Ba Duan Jin form. You can also do this exercise while seated.

❶ Sit comfortably with a straight back and make sure your entire body is relaxed.

❷ Clench your hands into loose fists.

❸ Tap your entire body gently with your fists. Start at your waist, then move to your back, paying attention to the area around the kidneys. Move to your shoulders (see illustration), down both arms, then to the front and back of your torso, and down both legs, finishing at your feet. Remember to be gentle—this exercise should be relaxing and enjoyable, not leave you with bruises!

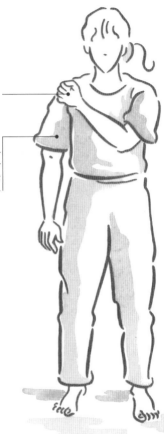

The fist you are tapping with should not be too tight or tense.

Tap gently over your entire body with your fists until you are thoroughly relaxed.

sensations you may feel during practice

As you practice qigong more intensively, you may feel sensations that at first appear strange. These can include tingling, warmth, itchiness, or feelings of an electrical current running through your body; you may see colors or visions. Your emotions may fluctuate from calm to giggly to tearful. These sensations and emotions are aspects of qi working in your body. They are natural, and you should try to let them happen without becoming attached to them.

You may also feel coldness, a cool breeze, or even pain, which could emanate from an old injury. These sensations arise in regions where qi cannot flow freely. They are signs that healing is taking place, though it is not complete, so you'll need to continue with your practice. Many practitioners find that a persistent ache disappears or diminishes over time. If you feel sleepy after your routine, it is an indication that your qi has some healing work to do, so you should rest and begin again another time.

Don't be concerned if you don't feel any of these sensations—it doesn't mean that your qi is not working or being improved by your practice. As you practice qigong more, your sensitivity will increase and you will begin to feel the sensations described here.

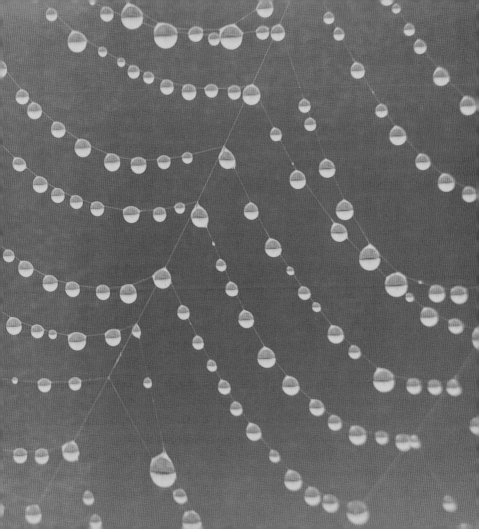

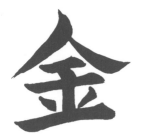 # meditation on metal

Buried deep beneath the earth, metal can be considered the basis of all other types of energy, the ultimate consolidation of the five elements. The energy generated by metal is an energy of strength, the bedrock of the life force. Metal energy is associated with the lungs, and so is essential to prolong life. Although humans can survive for days without food or water, you would die immediately if you stopped taking in breath via the lungs.

Because of this association of metal with the lungs, performing the Meditation on Metal can be especially useful for people who suffer from respiratory problems, such as bronchitis, asthma, or emphysema. People who are sad, depressed, or grieving can also greatly benefit from performing this meditation.

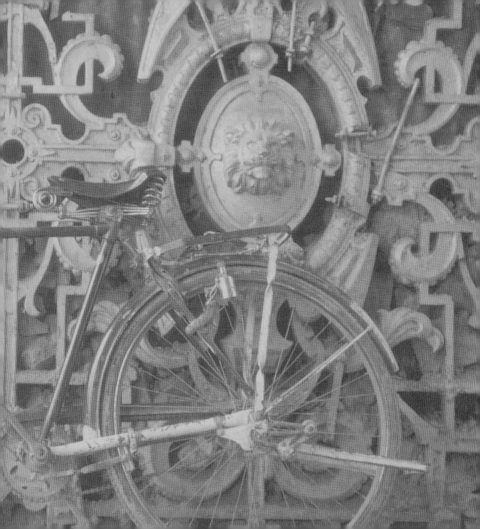

❶ You can do this meditation either indoors or out. If you meditate inside, have a window open to allow the elements into the room from the outdoors.

❷ Sit with your back straight; relax your body in the usual manner, relaxing individual parts of your body in turn from the toes upward.

❸ Visualize a giant shiny metal mountain in front of you; alternatively, imagine that you are surrounded by sheets of gleaming metal or that you are sitting on glistening metal. Whatever you do, always visualize the metal as being bright and shiny, not tarnished.

❹ Remain in this position for a while and try to feel the energy of the metal. Is it warm or cold? Does it make a ringing sound if you touch it?

❺ As with the other meditations, breathe the metal energy into your body; feel it filling up your lungs with its healing powers. Breathe out negative energy, expelling it from your body. Repeat this breathing exercise in cycles of 9 until you reach a total of 36 cycles, or as long as you feel is necessary.

❻ When you are fully relaxed, let your mind rest free of any thoughts. If thoughts come, let them go, and bring your mind back to nothingness, to your breath, or to the shiny metal that you are imagining is around you. Remain in this state for a few minutes.

❼ When you are ready to come out of the meditation, rub your hands together and gently brush down your body. You should now be feeling energized and refreshed.

introducing yi jin jing

The Yi Jin Jing (Sinew Transforming Exercise) form of qigong was developed by the Bodhidharma at the Shaolin Temple on China's Song Mountain. The routines, which were designed to help monks in their meditation, are now among China's most popular exercises. Like Ba Duan Jin, Yi Jin Jing aims to balance yin and yang energies and calm the mind. It does this through stretches for the tendons (sinews) coordinated with the breath; it also acts on the meridians to enhance the flow of qi.

the nature of
yi jin jing exercises

Yi Jin Jing exercises are gentle but require concentration. Visualization and focused attention on the breath are used to direct the mind and coordinate movements. The exercises are suitable for people of all ages, but they are particularly beneficial for growing children. Yi Jin Jing exercises also exert a powerful healing effect, particularly for chronic diseases.

Using the abdominal muscles for breathing is an essential part of Yi Jin Jing. This technique has the added benefit of strengthening the abdomen, which is used for breathing in two ways. During inhalation, you either contract the abdomen and expand the chest or expand the abdomen and contract the chest.

As you practice Yi Jin Jing exercises, let your body tell you how far to push it. The exercises sound simple and easy, but they do require strength. Periodically check your body to make sure it isn't becoming tense. You may find that your shoulders rise up or your hips stiffen; be mindful of such changes and gently coax tense areas to relax. Slowly build up the time that you are able to stay in each posture. Above all, do not rush.

the meridians

In the same way that blood flows through arteries and veins, qi flows through the body via pathways called meridians. These meridians, which are invisible to the eye, can be perceived with spiritual vision. Meridians can become blocked as a result of inharmonious living or disease, resulting in stagnation in the flow of qi around the body.

The meridians consist of 12 conduits (the Twelve Major Meridians) that link the internal organs; qi circulates among them in a specified sequence. In the west they are known by the names of the organs: the Lung Meridian, the Heart Meridian, and so on. There are also 8 auxiliary channels (the Eight Extraordinary Meridians or the Eight Miraculous Meridians), including the Du and Ren Channels mentioned in the discussion of the Dan Tians (see page 39). The Du channel runs up the spine and the Ren channel runs up the front of the body. Also, there are 15 smaller, collateral channels which have, primarily, a connecting function. The various meridians form a web that links the entire body and circulates nourishing qi to each part.

In acupuncture and acupressure, the flow of qi is regulated by placing a needle (in the case of acupuncture) or pressure (in the case of acupressure) at certain points on the meridians.

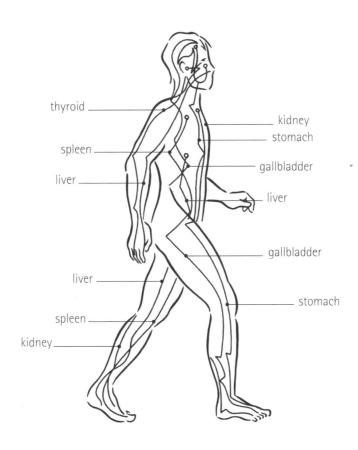

thyroid

spleen

liver

liver

spleen

kidney

kidney

stomach

gallbladder

liver

gallbladder

stomach

month9

Without going out of your door, you can know
the ways of the world.
Without peeping through your window, you can
see the way of Heaven.
The further you go, the less you know.
Thus, the Sage knows without traveling,
Sees without looking,
And achieves without ado.

From the *Tao Te Ching*

contents:

Qigong exercises help you achieve the deep-rooted stability and strength of a tree.

The ninth month is a time of turning our attention to other things. The garden has been put to bed, the harvest put up for the coming winter. Similarly, this month turns your attention to another school of qigong—Yi Jin Jing.

In order to stand tall and majestic, a tree needs roots to anchor it to the earth. You, too, can learn how to stand as rooted as a tree, using your body and mind to ground you. With the Yi Jin Jing exercises to calm your thoughts and strengthen your body, you will be prepared for further spiritual transformations.

This chapter features the first three of twelve Yi Jin Jing forms, which can be practiced in any order. These exercises will each give you the following life-changing health benefits: Yi Jin Jing Form One is good for strengthening your entire body, relaxing your mind, and increasing your sensitivity to the energy movements within and around your body. Yi Jin Jing Form Two provides a good stretch for your arms and upper body. Yi Jin Jing Form Three increases the harmony between your body and your mind and enables you to feel more alert.

The Meditation on the Breath, a very powerful tool, will help you further concentrate your mental energies. You will also learn to watch your mind, and so gain a greater insight into your nature. These meditation techniques, coupled with the other meditations featured throughout the book, will help you feel more confident both within yourself and in the world outside you.

In this month there is also a detailed discussion on the Taoist thinking that forms a philosophical background to qigong, including information on the nature of the twin principles of yin and yang, whose balance has its effect in every aspect of the universe, including your own body. There is also a useful chart that shows the properties associated with yin and yang.

yi jin jing form one

❶ Stand up straight with your feet shoulder-width apart. Your knees should be slightly bent. Try to keep your feet parallel, as if you were standing on train tracks.

❷ Raise your arms in front of you, as if you were carrying an enormous ball (see illustration). Your hands should be spread flat, with your palms toward you and your fingers slightly apart. Keep your arms rounded. Your body should now feel like a great sturdy tree with roots going deep into the ground, holding you steady and immovable.

❸ Look straight ahead of you. Clear your mind. If thoughts come, let them go. Be sensitive to the energies and emotions you feel. Stand in this position for 2 to 10 minutes.

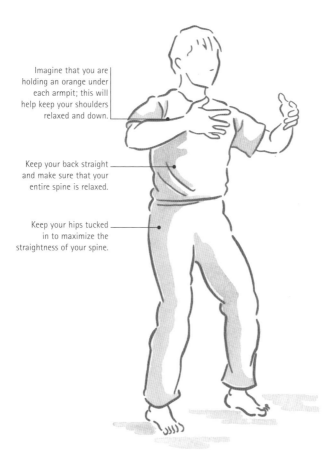

Imagine that you are holding an orange under each armpit; this will help keep your shoulders relaxed and down.

Keep your back straight and make sure that your entire spine is relaxed.

Keep your hips tucked in to maximize the straightness of your spine.

yi jin jing form two

❶ Stand up straight with your feet shoulder-width apart. Your knees should be slightly bent. Grip the ground with your toes. Feel that you have roots coming out of your toes and going deep into the ground, anchoring you in place.

❷ Open your hands, palms down, and raise them to shoulder level to form a T (see illustration).

❸ Relax your shoulders, neck, arms, spine, and hips. When you first practice this exercise, you may find that you have to remind your body (particularly your upper body) to relax.

❹ Lower your eyes and breathe naturally. Clear your mind, keeping it calm and relaxed.

❺ Stay in this position for between 2 to 10 minutes.

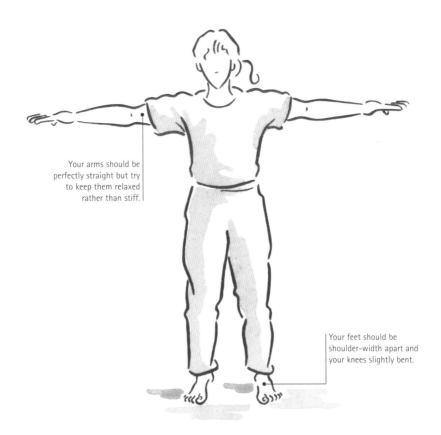

Your arms should be perfectly straight but try to keep them relaxed rather than stiff.

Your feet should be shoulder-width apart and your knees slightly bent.

yi jin jing form three

❶ Stand up straight with your feet shoulder-width apart. Your knees should be slightly bent. Grip the ground with your toes. Feel that you have roots coming out of your toes and going deep into the ground, anchoring you in place.

❷ Raise both your arms above your head. Interlace your fingers with your thumbs sticking out and push your palms toward the heavens (see illustration).

❸ Look at your hands, and then at the heavens.

❹ Lift up your heels slightly.

❺ Touch the tip of your tongue to your upper palate just behind your teeth. This ensures that your internal energy can move freely around your body.

❻ Clear your mind and be sensitive to your energies. Hold this posture for 2 to 10 minutes. After a while, your mind will be more alert and your body will feel completely whole.

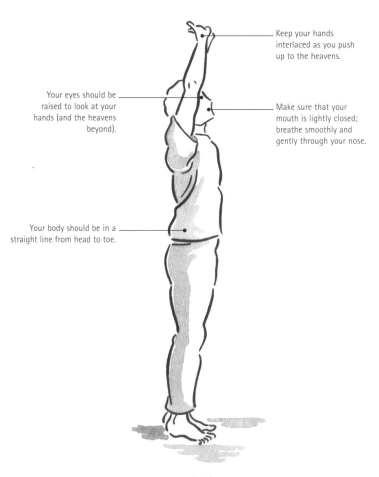

Keep your hands interlaced as you push up to the heavens.

Your eyes should be raised to look at your hands (and the heavens beyond).

Make sure that your mouth is lightly closed; breathe smoothly and gently through your nose.

Your body should be in a straight line from head to toe.

meditation on the breath

One of the most popular forms of meditation utilizes the breath as an object of concentration. You used this technique to a limited extent when you practiced abdominal breathing (see pages 26, 40, and 56). In Meditation on the Breath, your breath itself becomes the object of meditation.

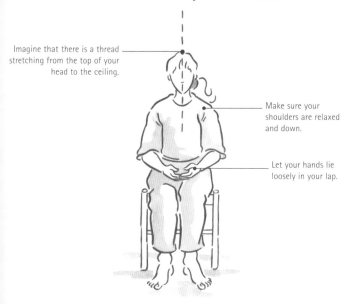

Imagine that there is a thread stretching from the top of your head to the ceiling.

Make sure your shoulders are relaxed and down.

Let your hands lie loosely in your lap.

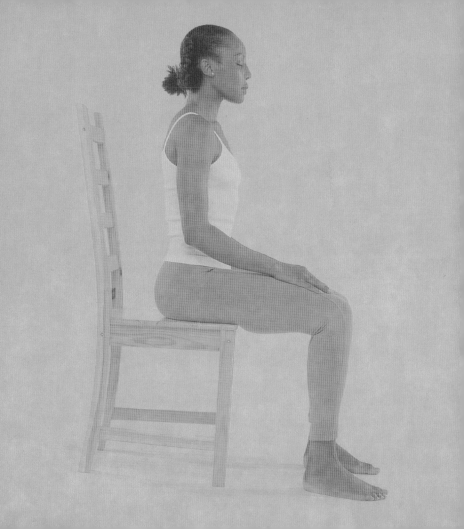

❶ Sit on a chair, positioned at the edge of the seat to ensure that your spine is straight. Alternatively, you may sit cross-legged on the floor. Lightly close your eyes.

❷ Systematically relax every part of your body, from your feet upward. To do this, bring your awareness to each individual body part in turn and tell it to relax.

❸ Now bring your attention to your breathing. Follow the breath all the way to your stomach. Let your breath take the lead, rather than trying to control its natural rhythm.

❹ Imagine each inhaled breath as consisting of golden light, a regenerating and revitalizing life force. Breathe into your stomach this way, repeating the process 9 times.

❺ Now direct your breath into your arms, first into the left arm and then the right. Again, imagine the inhaled breath as golden light. Concentrate on the center of the corresponding palm as you inhale—this will guide your breath to that arm. Perform 9 breathing cycles, each consisting of one inhalation and one exhalation, for each arm.

❻ Now bring your attention to your legs, breathing the same golden light into each leg. As you inhale, focus your awareness on the sole of your left foot. Perform 9 breathing cycles, then repeat the process on the right foot.

❼ Continue to follow your breathing, but now simply keep your attention on your nostrils. Perform 9 breathing cycles. Your whole body should now feel completely relaxed.

taoism

Underlying qigong and much of Chinese thinking and practice is Taoism. Many Westerners have only a vague notion of Taoism; even the Chinese have some difficulty in agreeing what constitutes Taoism. Some regard it as a religion, others as a philosophy, others as a set of healing practices. The word Tao translates as "The Way" or "The Path," meaning not just the way to achievement but the way of the cosmos. Taoism is the way to a harmonious understanding of the mind and the universe.

In Taoism, each person is seen as a microcosm of the universe. Patterns that occur in society or within the human organism reflect larger patterns in the cosmos. Taoists believe that observable changes in the universe can be studied; that knowledge can then be applied to corresponding changes within the body or within society. Thus, abstract Taoist beliefs form the basis for highly practical arts that guide and heal all aspects of human life. Taoism underlies qigong, forms of meditation, martial arts, astrology, feng shui, Chinese medicine and dietary science, and even military strategy.

wu ji and qi

In Taoism, the absolute beginning is called Wu Ji, which means absolute nothingness. What first emerges out of nothingness is qi —energy. Qi is the energy that drives the stars, the planets, and all matter; it is also the energy that gives life. This vital, life-giving energy is at the core of qigong.

The Tao gives birth to One.
One gives birth to yin and yang.
Yin and yang give birth to all things.

The complete whole is also part of the whole.
So also is any part the complete whole.

But forget about understanding and harmonizing
*   and making all things one.*
The universe is already a harmonious oneness;
*   just realize it.*

from the *Hua Hu Ching*

yin and yang

Qi is manifested through the two opposing principles of yin and yang. Yin means "the shady side of the mountain" and yang means "the sunny side of the mountain." Yin is associated with female energy, earth, darkness, coldness, dampness, and quiescence. Yang is associated with male energy, heaven, brightness, heat, dryness, and activity.

Yin and yang cannot exist independently—they are like the north and south poles of a magnet, like the front and back of an object. This interdependence is called tai ji, or "the highest." Everything contains both yin and yang, and all changes in the universe occur through transitions between yin and yang. Nothing is entirely yin or entirely yang, but sometimes, when there is disharmony in the universe, there is an imbalance of one over the other.

As far as the body and its functioning goes, a balance of yin and yang leads to health, an imbalance leads to disease. Yin is related to underfunctioning and weakness (such as cold hands and feet), while yang is associated with overfunctioning and excess (such as fever and swelling).

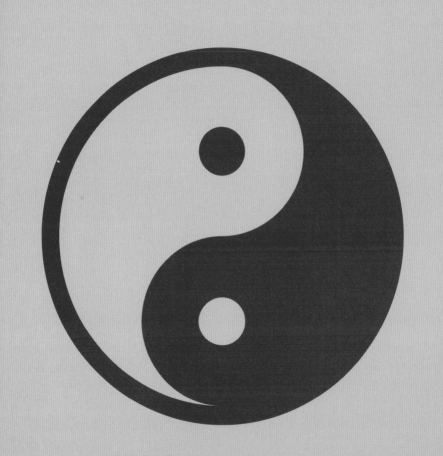

yin and yang properties and manifestations

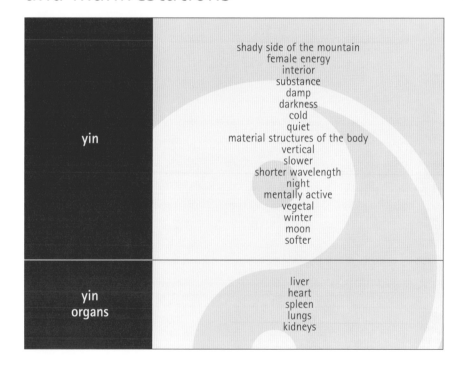

yin	shady side of the mountain female energy interior substance damp darkness cold quiet material structures of the body vertical slower shorter wavelength night mentally active vegetal winter moon softer
yin organs	liver heart spleen lungs kidneys

yang	sunny side of the mountain male energy exterior form dryness light warmth activity functions of the body horizontal faster longer wavelength day physically active animal summer sun harder
yang organs	gallbladder small intestine large intestine stomach urinary bladder

yin and yang properties and manifestations

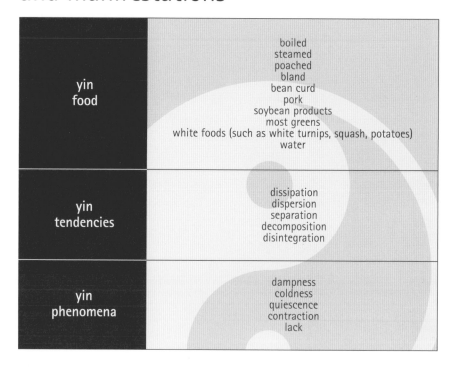

yin food	boiled steamed poached bland bean curd pork soybean products most greens white foods (such as white turnips, squash, potatoes) water
yin tendencies	dissipation dispersion separation decomposition disintegration
yin phenomena	dampness coldness quiescence contraction lack

yang food	deep-fried roasted stir-fried spicy and sour beef chicken eggs green peppers red foods (such as beans, peppers, tomatoes) wine
yang tendencies	organization assimilation gathering composition integration
yang phenomena	dryness heat activity growth excess

winter

fulfillment

At the end of the fall, after a period of conscientious learning and practice, you can allow yourself to rest on your laurels for a time and congratulate yourself on what you have achieved. You will find you have learned more about your body and mind, and that life has become calmer, easier. You will have become more in tune with your environment. Just as one season's end flows smoothly into the next season's beginning, your mind and body have become stronger and rejuvenated, ready to start the cycles of another season again, though now at a higher, wiser level.

month 10
month 11
month 12

month 10

The five colors blind the eye.
The five tones deafen the ear.
The five flavors cloy the palate.
Racing and hunting madden the mind.
Rare goods tempt men to do wrong.
Therefore, the Sage takes care of the belly,
   not the eye.
He prefers what is within to what is without.

from the *Tao Te Ching*

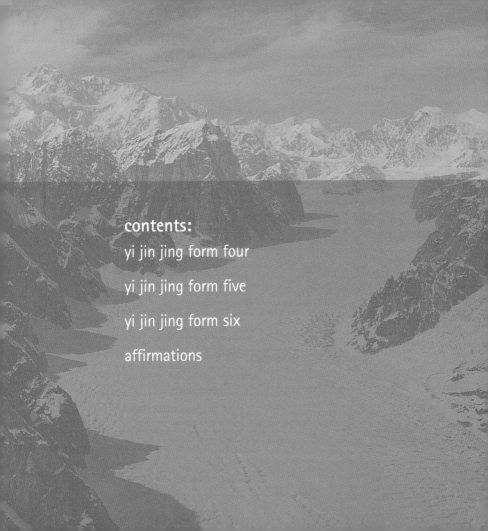

contents:

Changing your life means affirming your goals.

The tenth month is a month of change. Vegetation dies back, animals prepare for the coming cold months, winter arrives. During the past nine months of qigong practice, your body will have become stronger and your mind calmer. In addition to the continuation of your physical qigong practice, you can now take another step, learning how to reprogram your own mind to enable you to make the necessary changes for a more enjoyable and fulfilling life.

This month you will be introduced to a further three Yi Jin Jing exercises. Performing these exercises will strengthen your entire body even more. You may now be able to hold postures for longer, though it is still important to be mindful of your body and its limitations and not push yourself too far.

Specifically, the Yi Jin Jing exercises featured this month will have the following benefits to your health: Yi Jin Jing

Form Four gives strength to your neck, shoulders, arms, and back. The turn of your waist in Yi Jin Jing Form Five helps to strengthen your kidneys and stomach and also opens the lower Dan Tian, increasing the flow of qi. Meanwhile, Yi Jin Jing Form Six is good for expanding the chest, increasing flexibility and strength in the shoulders and arm muscles, and improving your concentration. If you practice this Yi Jin Jing form in the Horse Riding Stance, as shown in the Ba Duan Jin exercises earlier in the book, it also strengthens your legs, thighs, and buttocks.

In this month you will also be introduced to the powerful technique of using affirmations to help you achieve your goals and desires. You'll be presented with examples of effective affirmations, as well as guidelines for generating your own personal affirmations. Using affirmations in conjunction with meditation will enhance the benefits you have already obtained from the qigong exercises and meditations, adding an extra layer of relaxation and mental well-being to the benefits you have already built up.

yi jin jing form four

❶ Stand up straight with your feet shoulder-width apart. Your knees should be slightly bent. Grip the ground with your toes. Feel that you have roots coming out of your toes and going deep into the ground, anchoring you in place.

❷ Raise your left arm above your head with your palm facing up, as if you were shielding the top of your head from the sun or rain. Tilt your head slightly backward and look at your left hand. Ensure that your mouth is lightly closed, and breathe naturally through your nose.

❸ Place your right hand, palm facing out, on your lower back (see illustration). Your hand should be flat and relaxed.

❹ Stay in this position for 9 (or multiples of 9, up to 36) breathing cycles. Repeat on the other side for the same number of breathing cycles.

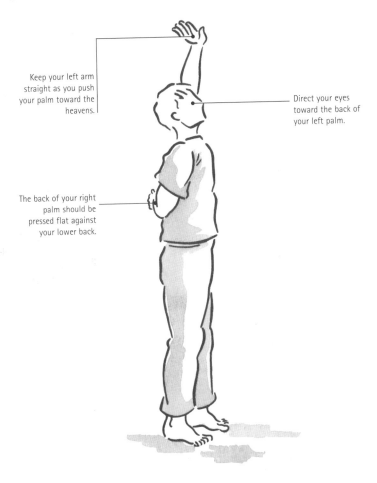

Keep your left arm straight as you push your palm toward the heavens.

Direct your eyes toward the back of your left palm.

The back of your right palm should be pressed flat against your lower back.

yi jin jing form five

❶ Stand up straight with your feet shoulder-width apart.

❷ With your left foot, take a step to the right, and then turn your body to the left. Point the toes of your left foot to the left, keeping them in line with your body. Your left foot should be pushing forward.

❸ Your right foot should be facing the same direction as your left foot but pushing backward. Lift your right heel slightly.

❹ Make a fist with your right hand and push it backward at waist level. Make a fist with your left hand and push it out in front of you (see illustration).

❺ Raise your left fist up to eye level, about 18 inches (45 cm) in front of your eyes, with the palm facing you. Look at your left hand. This position creates a nice sideways stretch.

❻ Your weight should be evenly distributed between your legs so that your center of gravity falls between your feet.. Let your qi sink into your belly. Breathe normally, with your mouth lightly closed. Maintain this position for 2 to 10 minutes. Make sure that your shoulders stay lowered and your upper body remains relaxed.

❼ Repeat the exercise on the other side for the same amount of time.

yi jin jing form six

❶ Stand up straight with your feet slightly wider than shoulder-width apart. A good way of getting the right separation between your feet is to initially stand with your feet together, then, keeping your heels together, rotate your ankles to form a V-shape with your feet. Now, pivoting on your toes, move your heels out as far as you can. Finally, straighten your feet so they are parallel.

❷ Bend your knees slightly, so that you are in a high Horse Riding Stance. Straighten your back, tuck your tailbone under, and make sure that your shoulders and neck are relaxed.

❸ Make fists with both hands and raise them to your sides, just above the hipbones. Ensure that you are breathing smoothly, evenly, and naturally.

❹ Exhaling, open your hands and slowly push them forward. Rotate your arms so that your palms face forward with fingers spread apart, and your arms are parallel. Look straight ahead (see illustration).

❺ Make fists with your hands again. Inhaling, slowly draw them back, rotating your arms to return them to their original position by your sides.

❻ Repeat a total of 7 times.

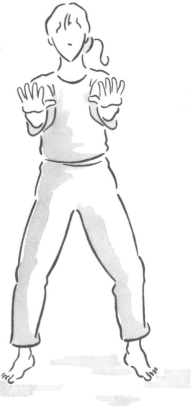

affirmations

The affirmation technique is based on repeating positive statements that relate to your problems or desires. You may repeat an affirmation continuously in any context, and then stop whenever you wish. The power of the affirmation will continue to work even after you have stopped saying it aloud. The most effective way to use an affirmation is to combine it with meditation, as follows:

❶ Sit comfortably, either in a chair or cross-legged on the floor. Your back should be straight; you may find it helpful to visualize a thread connecting the top of your head to the ceiling. Tuck in your chin slightly—this will help straighten your back.

❷ Close your eyes. Systematically relax every part of your body, as described in the Meditation on the Breath (see page 180).

❸ Bring your attention to the point between your eyebrows, your third eye, and hold it there for at least 5 minutes.

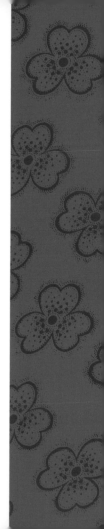

4 Now repeat your affirmation so that it is barely audible. Do this for another 5 minutes.

5 Next, repeat the affirmation mentally, without moving your lips, for another 5 minutes.

6 If you feel tired, stop repeating the affirmation and rest in a thoughtless state. If thoughts arise, repeat the affirmation silently.

You can practice this technique for a long or short time, according to your needs. If you practice regularly over a long period, you will find that it takes less and less time during each session for you to reach a deeply relaxed and tranquil state.

If you have spent time practicing such affirmations as "All is well" and "I am calm," you will find almost instant relief when you begin reciting these affirmations at a moment of difficulty. Even if you have not yet invested sufficient time in an affirmation, repeat it for a few minutes. This should bring some relief.

affirmations: examples

Here are some examples of suitable affirmations. You may use these if they apply to your situation or create your own affirmations, tailoring them to the particular challenges you face. If you do decide to create your own affirmation, try to use only positive words. For example, an affirmation of health should be "I am healthy" rather than "I am not sick."

for health problems

Two good general affirmations are:
- I am healthy.
- I am well.

If you suffer from specific health problems, for example of the lungs or heart, you could use:
- My lungs are healthy.
- My heart is healthy.

When saying the affirmation, try to visualize your lungs, heart, or other troublesome part of your body as being healthy, or visualize yourself doing whatever you think seems impossible or difficult to accomplish.

for relationship problems

If you have a problem in your relationship with person X, the following affirmations may be helpful:

- I am happy with X.
- X and I understand one another.

To make such affirmations more powerful, visualize you and person X hugging or reaching a mutual understanding.

for financial problems

If you are worried about your finances, you could visualize being surrounded by what you most need. Try the following affirmations:

- I have abundance.
- All will be well.
- The future is always bright.

for problems at work

If you are having problems with your career or are suffering from work-related stress, you could affirm:

- It will pass.
- I am a successful person.

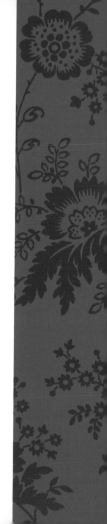

for stress or difficulty relaxing

If you are anxious or find it difficult to unwind, try lying down with your hands on your abdomen and affirming:

- I am calm, calm, calm.
- Peace, peace, peace.

for insomnia

If you have problems falling asleep because you are worrying about something or your mind is very active, try affirming:

- All is well.
- I am at rest.

The secret of success with affirmations lies in practice. You can practice affirmations anywhere—while driving to work, taking a shower, or doing housework. You could try writing out your affirmations on sticky notes and posting them in prominent places around your home.

To make your affirmations more effective, however, it is worth practicing them while you are in a meditative state, though practicing them as you do your daily tasks is much better than not practicing at all.

month 11

The highest form of goodness is like water.
Water knows how to benefit all things without
   striving for them.
It stays in places loathed by all men. Therefore,
   it comes near the Tao.
In choosing your dwelling, know how to keep to
   the ground.
In cultivating your mind, know how to be gentle
   and kind.
In speaking, know how to keep your words.
In governing, know how to maintain order.
In transacting business, know how to choose
   the right moment.

from the *Tao Te Ching*

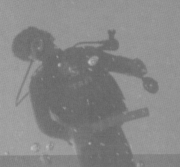

contents:

Plunging into the depths of consciousness, anything is possible.

The eleventh month is a time of turning inward, as animals withdraw from the outside world and burrow in for the winter. Likewise, as the weather becomes colder, people feel the need to stay indoors where it is cozy. Just as the body seeks interior spaces to keep safe and warm, at this time of the year the mind often delves into a time of reflection on the inner self.

The Yi Jin Jing exercises for the eleventh month are all aimed at strengthening the back and kidneys. This will give you more energy, as well as a deep inner sense of courage to help you to achieve your goals. Also, each of these Yi Jin Jing exercises has the following specific benefits. Jin Jing Form Seven is useful for improving the circulation in the chest, arms, and hands. It is a boon to

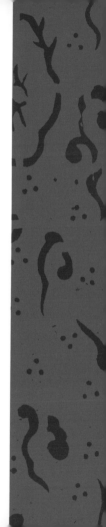

those with sprains in their hands and fingers, as well as to those who suffer from cold hands. Yi Jin Jing Form Eight strengthens the kidneys and the leg and back muscles. Yi Jin Jing Form Nine, with its sideways stretch, can be particularly good for preventing and relieving backache.

This month features two meditations that link the mind's two levels: the conscious and the subconscious. The subconscious mind lies deeper than the conscious mind, and it is the repository of feelings and fears that may normally be out of reach. You can significantly improve your outlook on life by using this month's meditations to help you penetrate your mind to reach the most profound depths of consciousness, effecting great changes in your life.

The Counting Meditation 2 is a different, seated version of the other counting meditation featured in Month 2. Practicing this meditation will enable you to reach a deeply relaxed state. You can then move on to the Meditation on the Third Eye, which is a great way to nurture your inner self, as it encourages you to delve within yourself to recall and visualize a scene that will bring you happiness.

yi jin jing form seven

❶ Stand up straight with your feet shoulder-width apart. Keep your back straight and look ahead.

❷ Now turn your body slightly to the right. Raise your right arm and rest the back of your head in the palm of your right hand. Pull your head toward the right.

❸ Rest your left forearm on your lower back. Make a fist with your left hand, palm facing out.

❹ With your right hand, pull your head further to the right, then relax. Be careful not to apply too much force. Coordinate your breathing so that you inhale as you gently pull your head and exhale as you relax your grip.

❺ Repeat the exercise 7 times in total, then repeat on the other side.

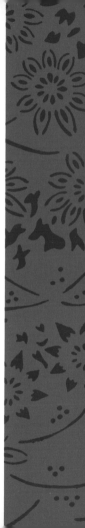

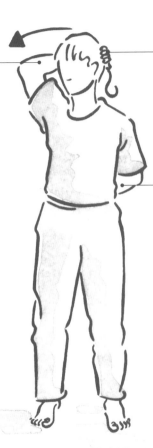

Gently but firmly pull your head toward the right.

Your right hand should be loosely holding the back of your head.

Rest the back of your left forearm against your lower back.

yi jin jing form eight

❶ Stand up straight, keeping your legs together. Take a step to the left and bend your knees until you are in the Horse Riding Stance. Look straight ahead. Turn your toes slightly inward, though not so far as to make the position uncomfortable.

❷ While keeping this position, inhale and exhale, making sure your breathing is smooth and slow. Breathe in this way for a few minutes.

❸ Lifting your arms upward, spread your hands out in front of you with your palms facing down and slightly above the level of your shoulders (see illustration). Make sure your spine is straight but relaxed as you lift your arms, and continue to look straight ahead.

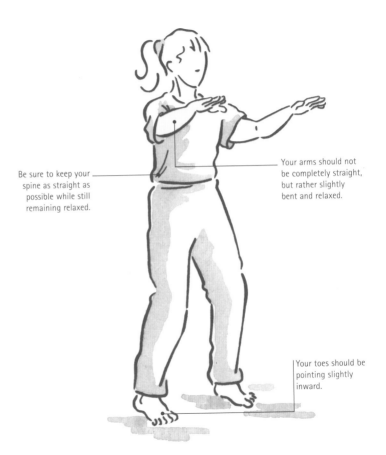

Be sure to keep your spine as straight as possible while still remaining relaxed.

Your arms should not be completely straight, but rather slightly bent and relaxed.

Your toes should be pointing slightly inward.

❹ Slowly and smoothly press your hands down toward the ground as if you were trying to grasp an enormous ball (see illustration). Grip the ground with your toes. Try to feel as if there are roots emerging from your toes, anchoring you firmly to the ground. Stay relaxed and make sure your torso stays upright.

❺ Now rotate your arms so that your palms face upward. As you do this, slowly raise yourself out of the Horse Riding Stance to stand upright and release the grip your toes had on the ground.

❻ Turn your hands again so that your palms face down, and then lower yourself into the Horse Riding Stance. Again, anchor yourself firmly to the ground through your toes so that you are steady and relaxed.

❼ Repeat the exercise 7 times.

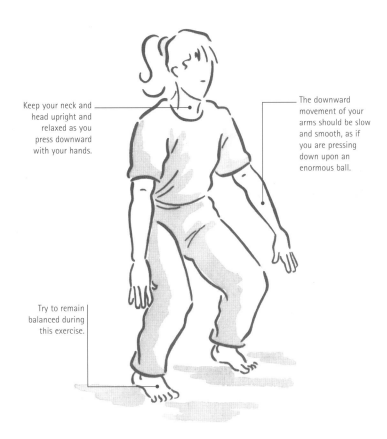

Keep your neck and head upright and relaxed as you press downward with your hands.

The downward movement of your arms should be slow and smooth, as if you are pressing down upon an enormous ball.

Try to remain balanced during this exercise.

yi jin jing form nine

❶ Stand up straight with your body relaxed. Look straight ahead. Take a step to the left so that your feet are shoulder-width apart.

❷ Make a fist with your left hand and raise it in front of your waist. Your right hand should be hanging down by your side. Spread the fingers of your right hand so they are not touching.

❸ While inhaling slowly, move your right hand over to your left shoulder.

❹ Continue to raise your right hand until it is level with your neck, then push backward with your hand (see illustration); exhale slowly. Turn your head slightly to the right and look to the right.

❺ Inhaling slowly, make a fist with your right hand and bring it down in front of your waist.

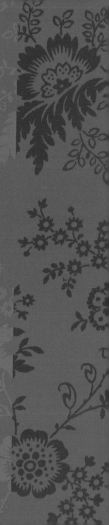

❻ Exhale slowly, opening your left fist and raising it over your right shoulder in line with your neck. Push backward with your left hand. Turn your head slightly to the left and look to the left.

❼ Repeat this cycle up to 7 times. Try to keep your movements and breathing smooth, natural, and coordinated.

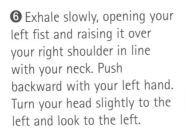

Be mindful that your body is relaxed throughout this exercise; periodically check that every part of it is loose and easy.

counting meditation 2

Here is another popular meditation method. It is based on the fact that concentrating on counting allows the mind to plunge into the tranquil depths of consciousness. The method is straightforward:

❶ Sit comfortably, either in a chair or cross-legged on the floor. Your back should be reasonably straight—visualize a thread from the top of your head to the ceiling to help you keep it straight. Tuck in your chin slightly to further straighten your back.

❷ Close your eyes to draw your senses inward. Count from 1 to 50, leaving a gap of one second between each count.

❸ By the time you reach 50, you will find yourself in a relaxed, deep state of consciousness. At that point, stop counting and enjoy the peace of this state. If thoughts come into your mind, simply count from 1 to 10. By the time you reach 10, you will have let go of the thought and you can again rest in a peaceful state, free from distractions.

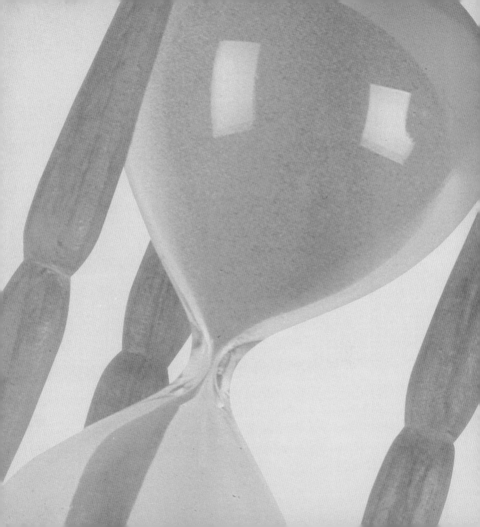

meditation on the third eye

The upper Dan Tian, often referred to as the third eye (see page 38), is our avenue to wisdom and intellect. It is through the third eye that we learn from our experiences and begin to put the events in our everyday lives into perspective, becoming clear-headed and open-minded. It directs our wisdom, judgment, intuition, intellect, and mental faculties.

The upper Dan Tian does not just govern the forehead but also the brain, eyes, ears, nose, neurological system, and pituitary gland. Because it is part of the hypothalamus, it can regulate body temperature and mood. A healthy third eye can see and understand more clearly, which makes it important to pay more attention to this vital part of your spiritual system. If you don't keep your third eye practiced and healthy, then you may become susceptible to irrational fear and depression. The mind will be slower to develop ideas and translate them into actions, and general understanding may begin to fail.

The following meditation is an excellent method of relaxation that focuses your attention on your third eye to bring it energy and nourishment.

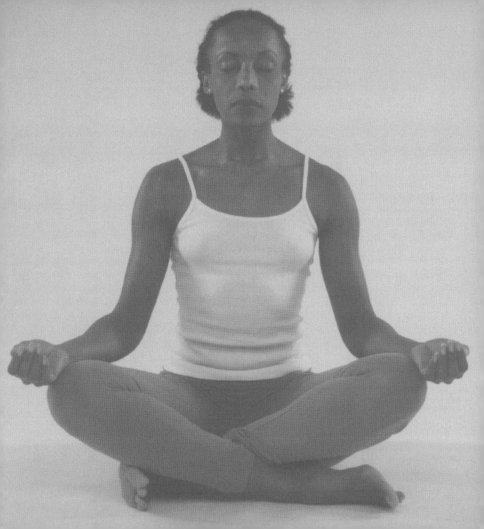

❶ Sit comfortably, cross-legged on the floor. Your back should be straight—visualize a thread from the top of your head to the ceiling to help you with this. Tuck in your chin slightly to further align your back.

❷ Bring your attention to the spot midway between your eyebrows, the location of your third eye (see illustration). With your eyes closed, hold your attention at this spot for at least 5 minutes. As your power of concentration increases with practice, you may feel some warmth or a tingling sensation in this area.

❸ When you feel relaxed, think of a time that you witnessed a breathtaking scene in nature or remember a wonderfully positive time in your life, such as when you first met your partner or when your first child was born. Relive the experience as

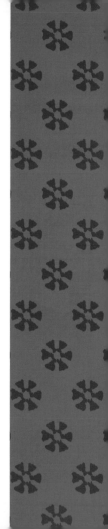

if you were watching it on a large screen at the location of your third eye. Try to feel that you are there again in that moment or place—breathe it, smell it, taste it, touch it, feel it, hear the sounds all over again. If you are totally absorbed in this experience, you may find that your face breaks into a smile.

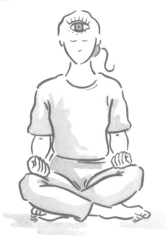

month 12

Nothing in the world is softer and weaker than water,
But, for attacking the hard and strong, there is nothing like it!
For nothing can take its place.
That the weak overcomes the strong, and the soft
    overcomes the hard,
This is something known by all, but practiced by none.
Therefore, the Sage says:
To receive the dirt of a country is to be the lord of its soil
    shrines.
To bear the calamities of a country is to be the prince of
    the world.
Indeed, Truth sounds like its opposite!

From the *Tao Te Ching*

contents:

Putting together everything you have learned, you now have the tools to fulfill your dreams.

The end of the winter is a time to look toward the renewal of the seasons, a time to fulfill your dreams. By using this book and making time to practice, you will find that your dreams can come to fruition.

The last set of three Yi Jin Jing exercises will again strengthen your body, particularly your back. As you have already learned, the back is a very important region of the body, since nerves from the spine branch out to many parts of the body. It is worth taking the time to familiarize yourself with these exercises, as they can prevent and relieve various back problems. The exercises are all good for balancing body and mind, and they have the following specific benefits as well: Jin Jing Form Ten, when practiced regularly, increases your body's strength and equilibrium. Yi

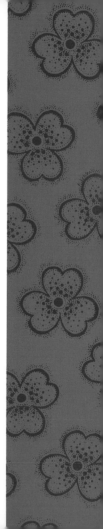

Jin Jing Form Eleven helps strengthen your back muscles, and Yi Jin Jing Form Twelve is good for relieving backaches, with the added benefit of toning your abdomen.

You have now been introduced to the whole set of twelve Yi Jin Jing exercises. The exercises can be performed in any order. Perform the whole set for a general sense of revitalization and well-being, or select individual exercises according to their effects on specific ailments. The Yi Jin Jing exercises finish with a closing form, which provides a great way to wind down and relax after performing the twelve main exercises. As well as being good for general relaxation, this Closing Form is good for the back and legs, improving circulation and therefore benefiting those who suffer from knee and ankle pain, sciatica, or lower back pain.

The final meditation in the book is a Meditation on Music. This one is enjoyable and relaxing—who doesn't love to listen to their favorite piece of music?—and its benefits are profound. It allows you to relax even further, calming your body and mind and enabling you to reach a state of heightened tranquillity.

yi jin jing form ten

❶ Stand up straight with your feet together. Look straight ahead.

❷ With your right foot, take a large step to the right. Bend your right knee and rotate your ankle slightly so that your toes point to the right.

❸ Extend your left leg behind you, keeping your left knee slightly bent. The toes of your left foot should be pushing backward.

❹ Lean your torso slightly forward.

❺ Extend both arms out to the sides with your palms facing outward (see illustration). Spread your fingers and press down toward the ground. Maintain this position for 9 inhalations and exhalations. Repeat the exercise on the opposite side.

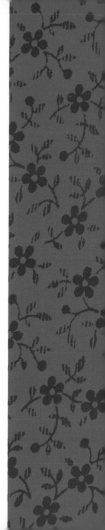

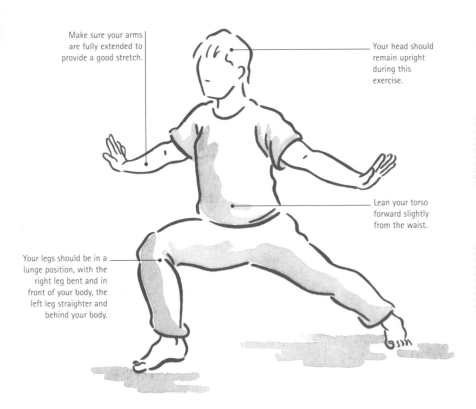

Make sure your arms are fully extended to provide a good stretch.

Your head should remain upright during this exercise.

Lean your torso forward slightly from the waist.

Your legs should be in a lunge position, with the right leg bent and in front of your body, the left leg straighter and behind your body.

yi jin jing form eleven

❶ Stand up straight with your feet slightly wider than shoulder-width apart.

❷ Raise your hands and place them on the back of your head. Your palms should be touching your head, your thumbs separated from your fingers, and the fingertips of both hands separated by a small distance (see illustration).

❸ Bend forward at the waist and lower your head to knee level. Keep your arms parallel to the ground with your elbows sticking out to each side. This opens up your chest.

❹ Lightly close your mouth and teeth. Place the tip of your tongue on your upper palate, just behind the teeth. This allows the Microcosmic Circle to flow around the body (see page 39 for more information). Do 12 breathing cycles in this position, and then straighten up into the initial standing position.

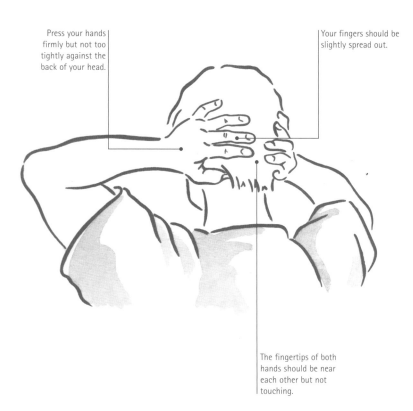

Press your hands firmly but not too tightly against the back of your head.

Your fingers should be slightly spread out.

The fingertips of both hands should be near each other but not touching.

yi jin jing form twelve

❶ Stand up straight with your feet together. Look straight in front of you.

❷ Move your feet as described in Form Six (see page 202), so that your feet are slightly wider than shoulder-width apart. Point your toes forward, as if you were standing on the two rails of a railroad track.

❸ Stretch out your arms and lean forward, pressing down on to your palms. Your palms should be open, with your fingers close to each other and your thumbs splayed out. Rotate your wrists so that your fingertips face each other. Your palms should be more or less parallel to the ground and facing downward.

❹ Keeping your legs and back straight, bend forward from the waist (see illustration). Your head should be erect. Look forward.

❺ When you can almost touch the ground, rotate your palms to face upward and slowly straighten up.

❻ Repeat this exercise 9 times.

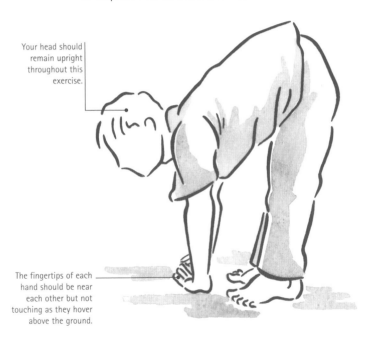

Your head should remain upright throughout this exercise.

The fingertips of each hand should be near each other but not touching as they hover above the ground.

yi jin jing closing form

❶ Stand up straight with your feet approximately shoulder-width apart. Look straight ahead. Make sure that your body is relaxed, your shoulders are down, and your back is straight.

❷ Let your arms hang comfortably at your sides. Your hands should be relaxed and your palms facing inward (see illustration).

❸ Lift both heels off the ground.

❹ Gently shake your body up and down 21 times.

❺ Lower your heels to the ground, and then stand still and relaxed for 30 seconds.

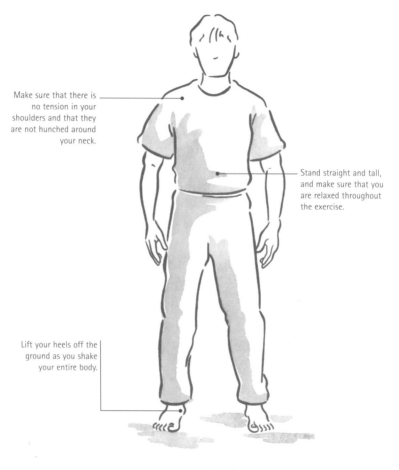

Make sure that there is no tension in your shoulders and that they are not hunched around your neck.

Stand straight and tall, and make sure that you are relaxed throughout the exercise.

Lift your heels off the ground as you shake your entire body.

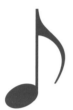 # meditation on music

Music can have a profound effect on both body and mind. Its ability to change your mood and help you relive past experiences makes it a very useful healing tool. Music also works well as a point of concentration for meditation.

To start your meditation on music, first choose a piece of music that you love. Ideally, it should be soothing and calming with no very loud passages. It is also important to choose a piece of music that you associate with good times and that makes you feel positive and happy. If there are any lyrics in the music, ensure that the messages are positive. There are many musical recordings available that are especially designed for meditation; you can use one of them, but it is not necessary to do so.

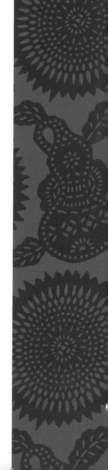

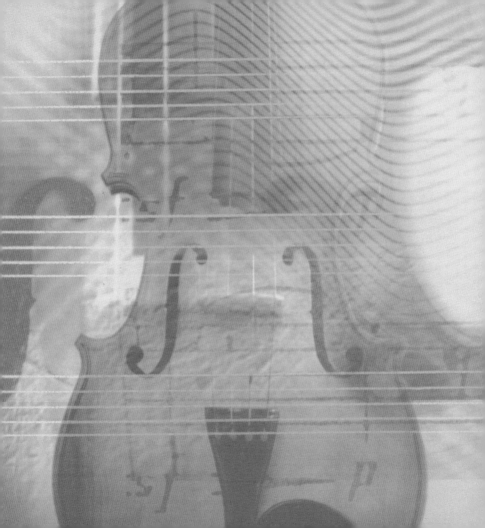

❶ Start playing your chosen piece of music at a low volume. It should be neither so quiet that you find yourself straining to hear it nor so loud that it forces itself upon you.

❷ Make sure that you are sitting comfortably, either on a chair or cross-legged on the floor. Keep your back straight.

❸ Bring your attention to the spot midway between your eyebrows—your third eye. With your eyes closed, hold your attention at this point for at least 5 minutes.

❹ Starting at the top of your head, gradually work down your entire body, ending at your toes. Pay attention to every muscle and joint, relaxing each part in turn. You should aim to spend about 10 minutes on this process.

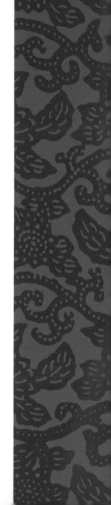

5 Now bring your attention to the music itself. Up to this point in the meditation, you will have merely been hearing the music in the background as you concentrated on your own body, but now try to really listen to it in the forefront of your mind. Be mindful of any emotions that it evokes. If your mind wanders, bring your attention back to the music.

6 Continue to listen to the music until it stops. Then sit quietly with your mind free of thoughts for a few minutes.

7 When you have finished your meditation, rub your hands together and rub your eyes. Gently tap your body all over, starting at your head and ending at your feet. This action helps release any toxins that have gathered in your body. You may now get up and enjoy the rest of the day.

moving on

Now that you have learned the qigong basics, it is time to put all your newfound knowledge together and move on to your own, unique qigong practice. You can formulate personal routines to relieve particular ailments you may have, or combine qigong with other sports, both Eastern and Western, to maintain a healthy lifestyle—for life!

creating your practice

This book acts as a starting point for you to incorporate a regular qigong practice into your everyday life. There is no set way to do this, and you don't have to perform all the exercises all the time. You can personalize your qigong practice so that it fits in with your personal needs and lifestyle.

While you are reading this book, learn the exercises at your own pace. Once you become familiar with the exercises featured in each month, go on to incorporate some of the exercises from the previous months into each session, combining them with the new exercises in any order. Repeat the exercises in cycles of 9 for Ba Duan Jin (see months 1 through 8) and in cycles of 7 for Yi Jin Jing (see months 9 through 12).You may combine two different types of qigong exercises in one session, or if you prefer, do one set of exercises in the morning and another set in the evening. Also, always try to incorporate some breath control into your exercise, or, alternatively, spend some time on the Meditation on the Breath.

When you have learned all the different exercises and practice them regularly, you will find, after a while, that you enjoy some exercises more than others. You can now go on to practice just the exercises that you enjoy most. One of the beauties of qigong

is that in many cases, the exercises you enjoy the most turn out to be the ones your body needs the most anyway. You can check this by referring to the "Quick guide to exercises for specific ailments" on pages 248-249.

In qigong, you should always incorporate a period of meditation into each session. Now that you have been introduced to all the meditations in the book, you may choose the ones you prefer and incorporate them into your exercise routine.

After this period of experimentation, when you have found a routine that suits you best both in terms of your health needs and your personal enjoyment, practice that same routine on a daily or regular basis. This will help you experience deep states of consciousness more easily. The mind and body enjoy and respond to familiarity and repetition; by regularly practicing the same routine, you assist your transition into a deeper state of consciousness, which is essential for healing the mind, body, and spirit. Take the time to practice, even it is for a few minutes each time, and you will find your body and mind gradually growing strong and revitalized. This can happen at such a level that profound changes may take place in your life. Most of all, enjoy your qigong practice.

quick guide to exercises for specific ailments

organ—ailment	ba duan jin	yi jin jing/meditations
KIDNEY • urinary and reproductive problems • lower back pain • problems with the ear • feelings of fear	• Holding the Heavens • Looking Backward • Looking for Hidden Treasure • Touching the Earth • Generating Waves of Energy	• All Yi Jin Jing forms, especially 10–12 • Meditation on Water
LIVER • hepatitis • gallbladder problems • conditions involving the eyes • feelings of anger or frustration	• Holding the Heavens • Generating Waves of Energy	• All Yi Jin Jing forms • Meditation on Wood • Counting Meditations

organ—ailment	ba duan jin	yi jin jing/meditations
HEART • circulatory problems • heart conditions • conditions involving the small intestine or tongue • feelings of hatred or cruelty	• Holding the Heavens • Looking for Hidden Treasure • Generating Waves of Energy	• All Yi Jin Jing forms • Meditation on Fire • Breathing Meditations
STOMACH • digestive problems • intestinal ulcers • diabetes • diseases of the mouth	• Holding the Heavens • Separating Heaven and Earth • Looking for Hidden Treasure • Generating Waves of Energy	• All Yi Jin Jing forms • Meditation on Earth • Breathing Meditations • Meditation on the Third Eye
LUNGS • respiratory problems • skin problems • conditions of the large intestine • feelings of sadness	• Holding the Heavens • Drawing the Bow • Generating Waves of Energy	• All Yi Jin Jing forms • Meditation on Metal • Breathing Meditations

qigong and tai ji quan

Ask a qigong master how many types of qigong there are and the answer might be two, a handful, or thousands. If you consider qigong very generally as the cultivation of vital energy, then there are literally thousands of self-healing arts that fall under the classification of qigong; one of the most well known is tai ji quan (t'ai chi chuan).

Tai ji quan consists of 108 slow, meditative movements that are full of intent. Some of these movements resemble qigong movements; others are quite different. Tai ji quan has several uses— as a means to spiritual growth; as a powerful martial art; and as a self-healing tool. Although tai ji quan makes use of qigong, it is fundamentally a martial art, whereas qigong is broadly concerned with the cultivation of qi.

qigong and gong fu

Gong fu (kung fu), like tai ji quan, is a martial art that requires the cultivation of qi. Qigong is also the basis for gong fu (and other Shaolin martial arts). Without training in the cultivation of qi, however, gong fu remains a rough, mechanical practice. One's internal power, which is related to qi, is the real power of a gong fu master.

qigong and sports

One frequently asked question is whether it is advisable to take part in sports while practicing qigong. There is no reason for you not to carry on enjoying the activities you participated in before you started practicing qigong. Of course, some of the qi that you have built up while doing qigong exercises and meditations will be utilized if you push yourself during a workout. Remember that, unlike aerobic activities, qigong exercises do not force your body to overwork, which deposits toxins in the cells that must later be removed.

Qigong practice can, in fact, enhance other activities—apart from increased suppleness and strength, you will have more energy to enjoy sports. It is up to you to find a suitable balance between qigong and other activities.

a note on chinese romanization

If you have wondered whether qigong and ch'i kung are the same, or what the difference is between tai ji quan and t'ai chi chuan, or how Peking changed into Beijing, you are not alone. Qigong and ch'i kung are exactly the same thing, as are tai ji quan and t'ai chi chuan. But note that the ch'i in ch'i kung is not the same at all as the chi in t'ai chi chuan . . .

The confusion is partly caused by the fact that translating Chinese into English is difficult enough, given the subtle relationship between pronunciation and meaning; things are made even more confusing by the existence of two systems for transliterating Chinese characters into the Latin alphabet. The Wade-Giles system, developed in the West, spells the cultivation of vital energy as ch'i kung, whereas the Pin Yin system, developed in China, spells it as qigong. Throughout this book, the Pin Yin system, which is gaining in popularity, has been used.

Pin Yin	Wade–Giles	English
Qi	Ch'i	Energy, vitality, breath
Gong	Kung	Practice, exercise, cultivate
Tai	T'ai	Immense, supreme
Ji	Chi	Ultimate, absolute
Quan	Chuan	Fist, boxing
Gong Fu	Kung Fu	Time, art, skill, effort

index